THE
EntreMD
Method

THE
EntreMD
Method

A Proven Roadmap for Doctors
Who Want to Live Life and
Practice Medicine on Their Terms

NNEKA UNACHUKWU, MD

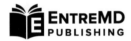

The EntreMD Method
*A Proven Roadmap for Doctors Who Want to Live Life
and Practice Medicine on Their Terms*

ISBN   978-1-5445-2581-5 *Hardcover*
       978-1-5445-2579-2 *Paperback*
       978-1-5445-2580-8 *Ebook*

To my fellow physicians...

The cavalry is not coming.

It is here.

It is us.

Contents

Introduction

"It's not how I thought it would be."

I've heard that sentiment hundreds of times from doctors over the last several years. We slog through a decade of hard academic work and grueling practical training to become physicians, then are deeply shocked and disappointed when reality falls well short of our original dream.

Most of us hoped that all those years of training would pay off through a meaningful life helping others. We anticipated all our sweat equity (and real equity!) giving us significant control over how we practice medicine, as well as job security and substantial compensation.

But the world of healthcare has changed. Administrators and insurance companies seem to be in charge of most of the key decisions. The list of what's being decided for us could go on and on, including things like how long we can spend with each patient, what medications we can prescribe, and how much time we can take off. The days when we were in control are gone.

Instead, physicians are often micromanaged and devalued by hospitals, corporations, and insurance companies. This has caused many problems, including physician burnout, which is currently at an all-time high.

Today, the majority of doctors don't work for themselves at all, and the ones who do often struggle as entrepreneurs.

But this book is not an academic study of how medicine has changed. We also won't engage in conversation about the rise of nurse practitioners, physician assistants, hospital-owned practices, or any of the other trends shaking up the healthcare world.

My focus is you, the doctor. I want to help you thrive in the chaos of the current healthcare space. I want to help you take charge of your career as a physician both inside and outside the exam room in a way that impacts a lot of people and also creates financial freedom for you.

What will change your situation is taking control of your career as a doctor by embracing entrepreneurship. That's exactly what the EntreMD Method is all about. I want to be clear that this isn't just a book for starting a private practice. If that's the kind of business you want, this is the right guide, but the principles also work for thousands of other business ideas. The concepts in this book apply to you irrespective of the kind of business you want to build, even if you're an employee wanting to build a personal brand. In the coming chapters, you'll learn how to create a business that allows you to do three things:

- Be in charge of how you practice medicine and/ or improve the lives of others.

- Create time and financial freedom for yourself so you're in control of your future.

- Do something that you love and that fills you with satisfaction, purpose, and meaning.

Does all that sound wonderful...but also a little "too good to be true"?

I know from direct experience that it is more than fantasy.

More than a decade ago, I began transforming from "just a doctor" to a doctor and entrepreneur. Eventually, the lessons I learned became the EntreMD community, created to support other doctors who are on the same journey. As the community has developed, it's been wonderful seeing other physicians take control of how they practice medicine and thriving financially, too.

Your journey as an entrepreneur will be worth it if you put in the work and follow the method outlined in this book. It's so satisfying to have a business that serves others, combined with financial freedom and the independence to practice medicine on your own terms.

WHAT YOU'LL LEARN

We'll start with a quick summary of the current state of medicine for doctors, and then I'll provide a general overview of the EntreMD Method to get you acclimated. Next we'll dive deeper, beginning with the mindset shifts you'll need to fuel your transition from disappointed doctor to fulfilled physician and entrepreneur.

Don't skip over the early chapters. You'll discover that many mindsets that work for a doctor won't serve you as an entrepreneur. Demolishing false mindsets and learning better ones is the foundation for the rest of the method. I'll also address common fears and misconceptions, including the idea that selling is sleazy and unprofessional.

Next, we'll turn to the habits you'll need to become a successful entrepreneur. You'll discover how daily habits are crucial to your success, and how to break through your comfort zone even when entrepreneurship gets scary.

If you're worried that you don't have the right skills to be an entrepreneur, I'll teach you how to learn them through the power of personal development. Or maybe you've already started a business and you've discovered you need better skills and habits to stop struggling and find success. This book will show you a proven method to do that.

After you've learned the right skills and habits, the last part of the book will focus on a blueprint that will show you how to go from idea to impact and profit. This is a step-by-step guide you can start implementing today. We all know they don't teach business at medical school, so consider this to be the MBA you never got. A successful business idea must serve others, but it also must be profitable. You'll learn how to analyze an idea to make sure it meets both criteria.

Of course, even the best idea is worthless if you can't communicate it effectively to your ideal client or customer. By the end of this book, you'll learn how to create a message that attracts the people you want to help and makes them eager to work with you.

The final step is to get the message of your business in front of as many people who need, want, and are willing to pay for your product and service as possible. I'll teach you how to amplify your message to create a critical mass of clients that can make your business wildly successful.

YOU CAN STOP
FEELING FRUSTRATED AND STUCK

Do I recommend that every doctor open up their own practice? I don't. That's just one possibility for an entrepreneurially minded doctor, and a path that worked well for me and others in the EntreMD community.

That's one of the best things about the EntreMD Method: it doesn't limit the kind of business you can start. If your dream is to open and run a successful practice, the principles in this book will help you do that. If your vision is to coach others to better health, or to launch a product that solves some other need, this method works for those business ideas, too.

And if you have no idea what kind of business you want to build, there's a whole chapter in this book to help you discover the right one for you.

The orientation of this book is meant to be extremely practical. It's a blueprint for effective action, not a dry study of business theory. All you'll need to get the most out of it is a sincere desire to transform your work life and reap financial rewards, plus a willingness to take action. I'll meet you in the middle with everything else you need to know.

To get the most out of this book, the first step is to be open to the idea that the changes in the healthcare field are actually an amazing opportunity for doctors. Many of us have been blind to that because we're trapped in an old vision of what doctoring is "supposed to be."

When you think like that, it's easy to get caught up in "doom and gloom," believing you have no choice but to stay frustrated and stuck. When you follow a proven method to start and run a successful business of your choice, everything looks different. You begin to see that there's never been a better time to combine your passion for medicine with the skills of being a successful entrepreneur.

Before we can begin to transform, we first need to understand our starting point. Chapter 1 is all about taking a clear-eyed look at the state of medicine today.

PART ONE

THE DAWN OF A NEW ERA

Why Entrepreneurship Is a Must

I t was the most ordinary of mornings when my life changed.

If there had been a video camera trained on me at that moment, nothing special would've been recorded. It was in 2016, and I was just sitting at my desk in my home office, preparing for the day. The earth didn't shake, a thunderbolt didn't suddenly strike, and no trumpets blared.

But internally, it felt a little like all those things had just happened.

The words that came to me were simple, but the implications were not.

"The way medicine has been practiced is gone…forever."

At the time of this insight, I had been running my own practice for six years, and it was doing well. But I still felt uneasy about the state of medicine. I hadn't been thinking in any kind of systematic way about the direction of medicine, but I also couldn't help noticing disturbing trends. It was bothering me more and more.

I also knew that very few doctors were facing up to the situation. When I talked about it, the responses were almost always things like, "We will always have jobs" or "The pendulum will swing back and things will go back to the way they used to be."

I wanted to believe the same thing, but the evidence for deep changes in the role of physicians was everywhere, and the trends were picking up steam. Looking back, I think up to that moment I had wanted to convince myself that there was a way around it all. That maybe somehow, someway, things would go back to a time when doctors had more control over how they practiced medicine and had more economic security.

I would describe that morning in 2016 as the moment when I let go of that fantasy and accepted that things had changed permanently.

I also remember thinking that the time was coming when it was going to get really ugly for physicians who didn't adapt to the new realities. The belief that physicians would have 100 percent job security—slipping away. The time when we had a virtual monopoly on practicing medicine—gone forever. The time when we could automatically expect to practice medicine on our own terms—that disappeared, too.

This insight should have shaken me up and depressed me. After all, I had just realized that the business side of medicine no longer worked for most physicians and that the trends were only going to snowball and become even worse.

But I didn't feel depressed. Not at all. I felt absolutely galvanized.

One reason I felt that way is because I knew that, if I understood a trend accurately, I could figure out the best way to respond to it. Instead of getting carried under by the wave, I could stay on top of it and ride it to greater success.

The other reason I felt so energized was because, in that moment, I discovered something about myself. It would take some time to figure all of it out, but I found out what I was supposed to be doing next with my life. Call it a mission, a vocation, a calling—whatever word you want to use. But I suddenly wanted to shout from the rooftops to other physicians:

"Medicine as we've known it is gone forever. However, if we can pivot and learn the skills we will need to thrive in the new times we find ourselves in, we can become better versions of ourselves. There is no cavalry coming; it is up to us to get back in the driver's seat and make our careers what we want them to be."

That morning I felt like a "knowing" came over me, and I suddenly had the certain conviction that the time for trying to hold on to a vision of the past of medicine no longer made sense. The role of a physician in the field of medicine would no longer respond to mild treatments; full-blown surgery would be required.

Maybe you've already had a similar "aha moment" yourself about how the field of medicine has changed permanently. Or maybe you're still clinging to the hope that somehow things will return to a time when doctors could count on complete career security and the ability to define how they practice medicine.

Whatever your current level of acceptance about the state of medicine today, it can be eye-opening to take a truly honest look at it. We'll spend most of this book focused on solutions, but it can help to have a deeper understanding of the problems first.

Let's start out with a basic level of frustration I hear from doctors all the time. The refrain usually goes something like this:

"I spent almost a decade to become a doctor. It cost a lot of money and I came out with a debt well in the multiple six figures. That's fine—I chose this path, and I knew the costs in time, money, and stress would be significant. But now I'm out in the 'real world' of medicine and it's nothing like I thought it would be. I can't do what I know is in the best interest of the patients and I feel like I'm on a hamster wheel. I can't be sure I won't be replaced, and I hardly have any time for family or friends or other things I love doing."

I can't help but sympathize when I hear stories like this. It's incredibly frustrating to pour your whole self into becoming a doctor only to discover the reality of today's healthcare landscape doesn't come close to matching your dream.

These doctors go on to tell me things like:

- They have no control over how much time they can spend with patients (fifteen minutes is often the max).

- Getting time off approved can be challenging and feels almost like you have to beg.

- Evenings are often spent charting instead of having quality time with family or simply relaxing.

- Insurance dictates a large part of how care will be provided.

It would be nice to say that all of the above are exceptions, but we already know that these are usually the rules physicians play by now.

One big trend is that doctors own less than half of all practices in the US. That's a dramatic change from decades ago when most practices were physician-owned. There is nothing to suggest that this trend will slow any time soon, because younger doctors are even more likely to work in a hospital-owned or investor-owned practice.

Hospitals and investors continue to aggressively buy up practices because it's profitable. Because the profit incentive is strong, it's not a trend that is just going to go away. And when doctors don't own the business they're working in, it's inevitable that they will have less control over their patient care, their time off, and their financial rewards.

THE RISE OF
NURSE PRACTITIONERS AND PAs

Another enormously significant trend is the number of nurse practitioners and physician assistants (PAs) in the marketplace. The truth is that MDs no longer have a monopoly on healthcare. And many hospital-owned practices are perfectly happy to replace physicians with less expensive nurse practitioners and PAs.

Stories like these are becoming increasingly common:

- Fifteen full-time physicians were fired in November 2019 from a health practice in the west suburbs of Chicago and replaced with nurse practitioners.

- In 2018, dozens of pediatricians working for a chain of clinics in North Texas found themselves out of work when those practices were taken over by new management. The explanation given was that the new management company favored a model that used nurse practitioners over physicians.

It's not unheard of for a hospital-owned practice to consist of one MD, with the balance of the staff filled out by nurse practitioners or PAs.

We could get into endless debates about whether this is fair, how much it impacts patient care, and several other topics. I'm not saying those debates aren't important, but in the end, the reality is it's happening. And it's not going away any time soon.

UNEMPLOYED DOCTORS DURING A HEALTH CRISIS?

In early 2020, the COVID-19 virus caught us all by surprise and forced massive changes to our society. Some were temporary shifts, and some continue to have a long-lasting impact to this day. One surprising thing in the healthcare world is that many physicians found themselves out of work, either furloughed or fired.

Think about that for a minute. In the middle of a historic health crisis, some doctors found themselves out of a job. You would hope that all physicians could be on the front lines, saving lives and helping people recover.

It's not my intent to say that there weren't many, many doctors who cared for people during the pandemic, in ways both heroic and ordinary. There obviously were. I also am not in any way blaming or belittling any doctor who did get laid off or fired during the COVID-19 pandemic.

My point is that up until recently, doctors assumed that their decade of education and training had earned them near total job security, as it always had in the past. But the global pandemic exposed the fault lines in the business of medicine. Some physicians found themselves collecting unemployment checks, and many others knew their jobs weren't secure.

All these trends—fewer and fewer physicians owning their own practices; the rise of nurse practitioners and PAs; insurance bureaucracy; and job insecurity and poorer working conditions—open up three paths for us as doctors.

One, we could stick our heads in the sand about it and hope somehow magically things will go back to a time when doctors had more control over how they practiced medicine.

Two, we could complain about it, becoming embittered that all that time, money, and sweat should've paid off more.

Or we could honestly face up to the changing state of medicine and use those insights to find ways to regain control of how we practice medicine, while also attaining financial freedom.

The first two paths are dead ends. Ever since that morning in 2016, I've been walking the third path. That journey has led to significant changes in my life. At the time, I was still working in my practice four days a week. I shifted to more of a CEO mindset and I learned more business skills I needed to keep my practice healthy and growing. Today my role is as the business leader of my practice, while still seeing patients one day a week.

The even bigger change since 2016 has been the amount of time I spend teaching others the EntreMD Method. Up until that point, I only knew how to doctor and how to run my practice. I wasn't yet a coach, and I hadn't done any speaking engagements or launched a podcast. I hadn't even thought of hosting conferences or retreats or starting a business school. Being the introverted introvert I was at the time, these were not even on my radar.

I decided it was time to embrace change, because I wanted to live a meaningful life helping others reach their dreams. I also wanted to be in charge of my future, including financially. I decided that doctors today desperately need to hear the message that there is an alternate path. We're not stuck and we're not victims. We can take back control of our lives and how we practice medicine.

The rest of this book is devoted to showing you exactly how to do that.

CHAPTER 2

The Paradigm Shift

Shaquille O'Neal was undoubtedly one of the best basketball players of his time, or really any time. The first overall pick in the NBA draft, he went on to win Rookie of the Year, and later an MVP award. He was selected for fifteen All-Star games, won two scoring titles, and was an NBA champion four times.

As impressive as all that is, none of that is what made "Shaq" fascinating to me. What intrigued me about him (and about many NBA players) is how well he understood that success was about more than what he did on the court.

Yes, he was a player, and what he did on the court was important to him—that's how he became a champion. But he also seemed to understand right from the beginning that he was also a business, and that he could turn that business into an empire.

He must have realized early on that building a business around himself would increase his satisfaction and enjoyment of life, and also help earn him even more money. He carefully built a brand around his likable persona. He did endorsements, became a brand ambassador, had his own show, and is now a studio commentator.

He then took that money he had earned for his work (what he did on the court) and from his businesses (anchored by the brand that he built around his persona), and invested smartly to build an empire. He reportedly used his wealth to invest in businesses like Google, which has earned him a very large, undisclosed sum.

What does this have to do with being a doctor?

I think that most doctors are stuck being players only. All their energy and focus go into what they do on the "court" (seeing patients, charting, navigating insurance, etc.). Looked at in one way, that makes good sense. If you trained to be a doctor, shouldn't you do what doctors do?

Yes, but if you focus on only being a "player" and neglect

business and empire, your ability to control your career and your earning potential is severely limited. You become more like the 60 percent of the NBA players who are reported to be broke within five years of leaving the league. I'm not saying you'll be poor in five years, but you're stuck in the same type of mindset as a player who never thinks about his brand, his business, or his empire.

When you focus only on your role as doctor, you are also stuck always trading your time for money. That should be part of your income, but you can't get the kind of leverage you need to attain financial freedom with the "time for money" approach. When you add business and empire, you'll be on a path to increasing your income exponentially.

My goal in this book is to take you from "just a doctor" to being a doctor AND an entrepreneur. And once you have a successful business, this can free up money for investing, which helps you on the way to building an empire.

Of course, I'm not in any way belittling a career as a doctor. It's a great thing to be. What I am saying is that we don't have to be one-trick ponies. There is so much more you can be, do, and have and I am challenging you to embrace it all. What if you didn't stop at one-third of what you could be doing? What if you did all of it?

You could see patients and do a wonderful job as a doctor. But you could also add in business and brand building skills. Those skills could be used to launch a private practice, and that's certainly not the only option you'll have. Maybe you'll add income from a new product you create, or from paid speaking, or from coaching. We'll talk a lot more about your options in Chapter 9, but the point to grasp now is that everything can change when you begin to think of yourself as more than "just a doctor."

This is also the cure for burnout—a common hazard for doctors, as we all know. Adding entrepreneurship to your original passion to help others as a doctor keeps things fresh and exciting. You'll never be bored. I've often told people that, since I started EntreMD, I haven't worked a day since. It's too much fun to call it work.

It's also energizing to increase your income and have enough to invest and start building your empire. This book will not cover investing or the specifics of building an empire, but I do want you to start thinking like Shaq. Don't get stuck playing on just one level. Add the other two levels and your satisfaction will go way up, both in terms of your impact on the world and your finances. On the other hand, if you stick to the level of an ordinary player ("just a doctor"), you leave your life up to luck or the whim of whomever you're working for.

Okay, maybe all that sounds great, maybe even inspirational, to you. But...how?

COMMON MINDSETS THAT
HOLD YOU BACK

More and more doctors are recognizing the need to take charge of their own financial future and sense of fulfillment in their work. They can also see that building a business is a path to do just that. But many are frozen at the starting line, unable to even access a beginning point.

Why?

When you're struggling to envision yourself as an entrepreneur, the problem is always your mindset. Our training and experience as physicians create mindsets that work against the mentality we need as builders of a business.

For example, as doctors, we fear failure, and that's a good thing. No surgeon wants to fail just so she can learn something from it. When it comes to medicine, we've rightly been trained in the mindset that failure is an enemy to be feared.

But an entrepreneur's relationship to failure is different. Failure is an expected part of the process. Too much failure is not good, but it's not an enemy in the same way it is in medicine.

Many doctors also have a knee-jerk reaction against any kind of selling. This is rooted in a misunderstanding of what sales actually is, as well as an inability to distinguish between good and bad selling.

These mindsets and several others keep doctors from making the transition to business builders. Until wrong mindsets are cleared away and replaced by healthier ones, no progress is possible.

That's why the first part of the EntreMD Method focuses on demolishing mistaken mindsets and demonstrating a better way. Chapters 3, 4, and 5 will show you how to do it.

HABITS THAT SUPPORT SUCCESS

Once a doctor sweeps away unhelpful mindsets, they need habits that support and reinforce the changes they want to make. For many, this will mean a substantial reorientation of daily habits.

It will also require a willingness to act in the face of being uncomfortable, and a commitment to personal development and learning new skills. If all this sounds a little overwhelming at the moment, I'll break it down for you in Chapters 6, 7, and 8.

If the first two parts of the EntreMD Method are getting the right mindsets and implementing the right habits, how do you then take what you learned and figure out what kind of business to start? And then how do you tell the world about it and make it profitable?

That's the final piece of the method, and in the last three chapters, everything will come together. You'll learn how to find and assess business ideas and then craft the right message for your idea, and finally how to get that message to the people who need your product or service.

I'm sure some doctors feel very unsure if they have a good idea in them. Others probably are thinking in very limited ways about what's possible ("the only thing I *may* be qualified to do is open my own practice"), and still others are coming to this book bursting with ideas.

Whatever category you fall into, I can give you ways to find ideas (or more ideas) to build from. Just as important, I'll show you how to analyze your idea to make sure it's viable, and then how to create a message around your product or service that will attract customers.

In short, the EntreMD Method will take you all the way from stuck to launching your business out into the world.

TREATING IT AS A HOBBY WON'T WORK

In the interest of being completely transparent, I do want to tell you that this method is for those who want to find a *profitable* business idea and then execute on it. As I like to say when talking to the doctors in the EntreMD Business School, we don't support hobbyists.

I want to help you find ways you can serve others while also making money. The idea is to both serve and earn. We'll go over more specifically how to do that in the last three chapters, but I do think it's important to know upfront that this is about starting a real business.

What many of my coaching clients and community members love about the method is that they get complete clarity on their messaging. When they post on social media, create a video, give a speech, or otherwise spread their message, they know exactly what they want to say. And it's not the old way of thinking about selling as something deceptive; it's communicating with clarity and passion about helping someone solve a problem.

"I WON'T HAVE TIME FOR THIS!"

No one today feels like they have any spare time. Between professional commitments, family duties, and some necessary downtime, it's hard for anyone to squeeze out time for anything else. It's true for everyone, and doctors feel the time crunch more than most.

It's true that finding time can be challenging. So I want to be clear that your commitment to building a business does not have to be full-time hours. Some business launches will be a full-time commitment (e.g., opening a practice), but for many businesses, three to five hours a week will be enough to get started.

As I said, you can't have a "hobbyist" mindset, but that doesn't have to mean you're required to put in full-time hours. Just like Shaq did, you keep playing on the court while also working in time to build your business.

The idea that "I won't have time for this" is similar to many of the mindset blocks we'll be overcoming. We look for ways to talk ourselves out of branching out. When you start slipping into negativity, I want you to think about this:

The overall acceptance rate for most medical schools is between 1 and 3 percent. One hundred people apply; one to three get in. You were one of those people.

You learned skill after skill. You can do delicate, difficult things like intubating a premature infant. If you're a heart surgeon, you can cut open a human heart and fix it. If you're an emergency medicine physician, you save people on a regular basis, many of whom are right at death's door.

And you're worried you can't do *this?* I'm not saying finding the right business idea is always easy, or that this won't require some sweat equity, but you've already proven you're equal to daunting challenges.

Now that you have a broad overview of the EntreMD Method, let's dive into the method itself.

PART TWO

REDESIGN YOUR MIND

CHAPTER 3

Mindset Myth #1: "I'm a One-Trick Pony."

I n 2010, I made what many doctors would consider a crazy decision.

I was only fifteen months out of residency, and I decided to start my own practice. Fewer and fewer of us are starting our own practices these days, and to do it about a year out of residency is pretty much unheard of.

To be perfectly honest, it was probably fair to judge my decision as foolish, at least at first. I was naive about what I was getting myself into. I was under the illusion that I could just hang the proverbial shingle and patients would fall over themselves to find me. That philosophy would've worked out just fine decades ago, but not in today's healthcare world.

After I launched, I wasn't attracting enough patients to meet my goals and I wasn't sure why. When I compared my practice to those that were successful, my frustration grew. Those practices had tons of fabulous reviews and beautiful websites, and appeared high up in online search results. Patients had to wait as long as two months to get appointments with some of these doctors, while I would have five patients show up on a busy day.

The successful practices came in different shapes and sizes—some were large and some were more boutique. But all the successful ones were sending out the right signals, and I could tell that they knew the secret sauce for a profitable and well-run practice. But what was that sauce? Maybe it was the right combination of hidden knowledge, natural-born business talent, and plain old good luck.

Whatever it was, I didn't seem to have it, and that was a little scary.

Okay, actually it was very scary. I had signed a three-year lease for office space. I had locked myself in contracts for multiple services like phone, fax, internet, insurance, and other expenses. I'd quit my job to take a per diem job at the local emergency department to keep money coming in while I grew the practice.

At the time, I felt exactly like a deer caught in headlights. What had I done? I secretly wished I could back out of the whole thing, but I knew it was too late for that. I had to make this work.

It was around this time that I began reading an excellent self-development book by Brian Tracy called *Eat That Frog*. It's packed with great advice, and there was one particular statement in the book that instantly transformed how I thought about building my practice: all business skills are learnable.

When I read that, I paused. Then I repeated it to myself.

All business skills are learnable.

In a flash, I realized that doctors with successful practices weren't better than me. They had been given no magical powers inaccessible to the rest of us, and it wasn't some talent they were just born with. I had placed limits on my thinking under the false assumption that these other doctors were better at this than me "and that's just the way it is."

The difference between the successful practices and my floundering practice was this: those doctors had mastered business skills. I didn't have those skills yet, but I could learn them. It was as simple as that. It wasn't some personal shortcoming or a lack of capability on my part.

The physicians who owned these practices knew about things like marketing, hiring the right people, leading teams, profit and loss statements, etc. In other words, they knew what they needed to know to run a successful business. That meant all I had to do was learn those same business skills. Would that be hard work? Sure. Would it take some time to learn what I needed to know? Of course. But now I knew it was possible for me to thrive. It was no longer out of reach for me.

Then a second insight came to me, one that made Brian Tracy's statement even more exciting. I recalled that no one is better at learning new skills than physicians. I'd spent a whole decade learning to become a physician. I slogged through thick books for long hours and sometimes took five-hour exams to prove that I had mastered the concepts. I had also spent hundreds of hours in intensive care units, general floors, and clinics to master practical skills. If running a great business is all about skill development, that was something I had already proven to myself that I had mastered.

I've also since discovered that I'm far from the only doctor who has struggled with these issues. I hear from doctors on a regular basis who tell me, "I'm just a doctor. I have no other marketable skills." Some others say, "I can't do anything else that can pay me like my clinical skills and I have student loans to pay off." For one, you probably already have more marketable skills than you think. But even if that's true at this moment in time, physicians should never lack confidence that they can learn more skills. There are very few professions that could match ours for the ability to learn new things.

Of course, I'm not denying that many of us doctors start off with an obvious skills deficiency in business. In the finance world, they refer to poor investments as "doctor deals." The implication, of course, is that most doctors are not savvy in the financial world and don't have the skills to confidently build successful businesses.

My point is that there's absolutely no good reason for us to *remain* weak at business. It's not like there's some part of the brain related to business that we're missing. It's only because of this mindset that we don't have business acumen and don't learn it. It makes no sense when you think about it.

The "I'm just a doctor" mindset is one of the most damaging limiting beliefs you can have, and it's the one that will stop you before you even get started.

I hear this expressed in many different ways:

- *"This is all I know how to do; I'm a one-trick pony."*

- *"Being a doctor is my only marketable skill."*

- *"It took me over a decade to become a doctor; I'm now set in my ways."*

- *"This is who I am; I don't know how to be something else."*

All these statements add up to the same thing. You've convinced yourself that you can't change and acquire new skills. Your first task on your journey to being an entrepreneur is to rid yourself of this mindset myth.

ACCEPTANCE

Imagine how you would react to a friend who told you she couldn't succeed because she's "just a doctor."

How would you respond? "Yes, you're right. You are just a doctor. You'll just have to accept your lot in life."

Of course not. You'd remind her of all she had already accomplished just to become a doctor. You'd remind her of her talents and her ability to learn new things, and you'd probably be able to come up with several other positive points given time to reflect on it.

Don't you have these same qualities and abilities?

To get rid of this limiting belief, the first step is simply accepting the truth. You do have the ability to control your financial future, and you can create a career and business that you love. Understanding and accepting this is hugely liberating—something I know personally and also have witnessed firsthand.

However, I've also seen this liberating insight evaporate when it's not backed up by action. I'll be providing a lot more specifics on action in the later chapters. For now, let's continue on to the next step: immersion.

IMMERSION

You need to immerse yourself in as many resources about entrepreneurship as you can on a daily basis.

Think of it this way: if you wanted to learn Spanish the fastest and most effective way, that would mean moving to Spain to create a forced immersion in the culture. You'd be hearing Spanish radio and television, all the signs would be in Spanish, everyone around you would be speaking it —you would learn it.

As a doctor with little to no business skills, you need to move yourself to "entrepreneurial land." You should be constantly reading books, listening to podcasts, watching quality videos, and using other resources that will expose you to the world of entrepreneurship. You will learn how entrepreneurs think, act, respond to challenges, and pivot. This process will transform you in ways you did not think possible.

It drives me a little nuts that some people seem to think they can read one book or listen to a handful of podcasts and that should give them enough knowledge to effect a complete change. Then when their lives of course don't transform in a short period of time, they decide, "This stuff doesn't work," or "I guess I'm just not the kind of person who can do this."

Immersion works, but it also requires consistency over time. I began this process eleven years ago and I've never stopped learning. It does work, and the longer you do it, the faster and bigger your transformation will be.

Learning the skills you need to be a successful entrepreneur won't take you a decade like it did to become a physician. But you can't expect to go from no business skills to successful entreprelneur without spending time immersing yourself in the business world.

ACCOUNTABILITY

The other piece of the puzzle for breaking this mindset is accountability. Even if you've accepted (in theory) that you can learn new skills, actually doing it can be scary. The first thing to understand is how incredibly normal this fear is.

I've been terrified during certain parts of this journey. My coaching clients and community members have had the same experience. It gets a little less scary when you realize everyone else has felt the same anxieties. But still, fear can stop us if we don't have the right accountability and support at the right time.

Many people think the best place to start is getting an accountability partner in either a friend or maybe a fellow doctor who wants to make the same journey. Now, I'm not saying you can't try that or that it won't work. I can only tell you that in my experience it's usually ineffective.

For one, friends are more likely to let you off the hook and not push you when you need to be pushed. That's understandable; you're friends. It's kind of like the difference between agreeing to meet regularly with a friend to walk versus hiring a personal trainer. Ninety-nine times out of a hundred, you're going to get in better shape faster with a personal trainer.

The other problem with inexperienced accountability partners is that they don't know what pitfalls to warn you about, nor how to help you get back on track when you need it. And you'll need it.

Hiring an experienced coach or joining a program can exponentially increase your business growth. Left on our own, most of us will dither and delay. With the correct guidance and accountability, most accomplish more in a month than they did in years on their own.

Nothing destroys a bad mindset more permanently than this kind of accomplishment. Action and success breed more action and success.

The right accountability partner can also help you with the flip side of the coin, and that's staying patient and not expecting success to happen all at once. There are a lot of submilestones on the way to bigger success.

Having structure and accountability to help you overcome adversity and stick with it can be the difference between ultimate success versus giving up. Having the right coach can help you maintain high expectations, and also make sure those expectations are realistic for the stage of the journey you're on.

So what happened to my practice after I committed myself to learning business skills? I learned there were no mysterious reasons they were profitable, no secret initiation that someone hadn't invited me to participate in. In about a year, my practice became one of those successful practices that I looked up to when I first launched. I also didn't have to waste any energy comparing myself to other "lucky" practices. That creates nothing but frustration, and sometimes even destructive emotions like envy. Now I knew it wasn't luck, and it all started with a mindset shift.

That shift meant that I now accepted that I could learn business skills, and that I could implement them in my own business to make it a success. Recognizing that I could respond to the changes in the world of medicine, and that I no longer had to stop at being a doctor, changed everything for me.

If you've struggled with the idea of "I'm just a doctor," I hope now you can see that as a false and limiting belief. Instead, accept that you can learn the skills you need to gain control of your future.

That's the good news. The bad news is that many doctors get past this mental block, only to stumble on another misguided mindset rooted in fear. How to overcome that is what the next chapter is all about.

CHAPTER 4

Mindset Myth #2: Fear of Failure, Fear of Success

In 2019, I decided I wanted to do my very first live event. Many people would have likely called this another crazy idea. Whether it was crazy or not, if I was doing it, I wanted it to be top notch, and I went scouting for a venue that would be perfect.

I looked at a well-known hotel space in Atlanta for hosting a one-day event. I was quoted a price of $10,000. And that was for just the space, not for food or anything else. My reaction was "TEN WHAT?"

To give you a little more context: at that point EntreMD was still in the early stages. I had a relatively small mailing list of two hundred people, and I didn't even have a website yet. I had been doing some one-on-one coaching but didn't yet have a formalized EntreMD program and community.

Once I was hit with a potential $30,000 bill for the event, including food, A/V equipment, and conference materials, I had the excuse I needed to change my mind and wait until I was "ready." Surely next year I'd be more comfortable and less fearful, right?

Here's a list of reasons I could have given for postponing the event:

- The cost is too high.

- I'm not ready: my mailing list is too small.

- I don't even have a website yet!

- By next year, I'll be a better organizer and better speaker.

I could have gone on like this forever. But all of that is the fear of failure talking. It's also a belief that if an event won't be perfect, you shouldn't try it. By then I had progressed enough in the entrepreneurial mindset to recognize this trap and avoid it.

If I didn't do it in 2019, then 2020 would be the same thing all over again. I'd find excuses why it wouldn't be perfect next year, too. I'd always dig out plausible-sounding reasons why it would fail, no matter what year I chose to finally do it.

In other words, I knew it would still be my first time if I waited until the next year. There would inevitably be imperfections that year, too.

So I made the decision to not give in to the fear of failure and find reasons to make this event happen even if it wasn't going to be at the perfect venue or be flawlessly executed.

My brother is the music director at our church, and he reminded me we had an events space at the church. Instead of handing a hotel $10,000, why not use a fraction of that money to make over the church space into a conference-style venue? That's what we did. I also found a financial advisor willing to sponsor the event, which paid for all the food.

My brother also said he would help me stream the event live for those who couldn't come in person. The upcoming event also motivated me to get an EntreMD website up and running. I started doing as much publicity as I could to generate some excitement.

On June 8, 2019, forty-seven doctors from nine different states attended my first event in person. People all over the US and in nine countries around the world watched the livestream.

Was it perfect? No. But people loved it and told me how much value it created for them. It advanced my business and taught me lessons for hosting future events. In 2020, the second EntreMD event registered 321 doctors from twenty-five states. The 2021 event registered 533 doctors from all over the world. Imagine all the lives that would not have been impacted if I didn't dare my fears and do it anyway.

THE FEAR OF FAILURE IS UNIVERSAL

I have a private Facebook group for the EntreMD community, and I require three questions to be answered to get admitted to the group. One of those questions is, "What is the biggest challenge you're facing in your business now?"

The most common answer is, "I don't know the next steps to

take." That's why this book exists, to offer people a roadmap that shows them the steps.

But it's also important to note the second most common answer, which is, "I'm afraid of failure" (or some version of that statement).

The people answering this question are interested enough in entrepreneurship to be asking to join a Facebook group on the topic. So they've already at least partially overcome the mindset myth from the last chapter. They know they want to add entrepreneur to their identity as doctors.

But then the next mindset stumbling block appears in front of them: fear of failure. It's amazingly common.

I can completely identify. For one thing, in my first year of owning a practice, I lived in terror of failing. It was so bad at the beginning, I refused to hire anyone because I feared I wouldn't be able to generate enough revenue to pay them.

If you think I'm exaggerating how much I feared failure early in my practice, let me tell you what I did instead of hiring people at the beginning. I answered my own phones under the pseudonym Ella. I took patients' vitals myself, and I gave them their shots. I was even the one who stayed at the end of the day to do my own billing. Talk about fear!

I hope this gives you some inspiration, because if I was eventually able to overcome all that, I'm sure you can overcome your fears.

The truth is the fear doesn't completely go away. I've felt this fear of failure all along my journey as I created a business around EntreMD. Despite that, I've been able to continue to press forward and grow by leaps and bounds. Perhaps if I share how I've come to think of fear's role in my business, it will help show you how to not let it stop you.

I spent most of my life being a fearful person: the fear of rejection of myself and my ideas, the fear others won't like me enough, an introvert's fear that I'll make a fool of myself when I get up on stage.

I'd look at outwardly confident and brave people and just assume they were given a gift I didn't have. I thought, "Wouldn't it be nice to be like that?" It's only with time I've realized almost everyone has the fear going on inside, and some are just better at moving forward in spite of it.

I had read things about courage not being the absence of fear, but the willingness to act in the face of fear. It made sense to me, but somehow it never sunk in. I continued to let my fears stop me.

One day, I reached the point where I'd had it with letting fear have so much power. I reflected that I had felt fear for a good bit of my journey to become a doctor, yet I became a doctor anyway. I remembered my anxieties as an entrepreneur, yet I was succeeding in business anyway.

I decided that if I couldn't completely rid myself of it, I wasn't going to let it stop me either. I talked to my fear: "Fear, since you won't go away, come sit down right next to me and watch me succeed."

Thinking this way now gives me a clear distinction between myself and my fear. It's almost like a separate entity. I can say, "You want to hang out with me, that's fine. I can't stop you. But you don't get to drive and I'm still going to do what I need to do."

The attempt to rid myself of fear was a waste of energy. It wasn't going anywhere no matter how hard I worked on my mindset or how much success I attained. Setting it to one side and doing what I had to do anyway was the solution.

DOCTORS AND FEAR
OF FAILURE

Doctors have more trouble than most with fear of failure, and for good reason. For one, if you decide back in high school you want to earn an MD, you better have a long track record of almost unbroken success academically, all the way until you earn that medical degree. As they say at NASA, "Failure is not an option."

This fear of failure gets reinforced all through medical training and continues throughout your career as a doctor. We've acquired a healthy fear of failure because we deal with life-and-death situations, and a certain level of accuracy will always be required.

But in the world of entrepreneurship, it's completely different. You don't want to harm your business, of course, but you also can't be so prudent that you never innovate. In business, it's fail fast, learn from it, and iterate quickly.

Doctors struggle to bring a different mindset to business, because we never want to "fail fast" on our patients just so we can learn a lesson or improve on the next patient. In the world of entrepreneurship, you obviously don't want to fail all the time, but you also recognize that failure is a part of long-term success. You do a speaking gig, and it doesn't go as well as you hoped. Unlike with patients, the audience didn't stay sick or die if you weren't successful. Instead, you learned something. And if you do it long enough, you'll stop failing and start seeing consistent success.

Past failures no longer matter because you got where you needed to be. This is why embracing failure is okay, even good, in entrepreneurship. It's going to happen as part of the process. If you don't embrace it, you won't be able to move through the process that leads to success. You'll stop growing.

What I find with doctors is that our fear of failure often leads to perfectionism. It's a huge trap for doctors. I can't tell you how many doctors have told me they can't launch their business because their website isn't perfect yet. There's always going to be something not perfect that will hold us back if we let it.

What do we do in place of perfectionism? Do we just say, "Whatever"? No. We focus on excellence instead of perfection.

Think of it this way. Perfect work means work without fault or defect; don't make that your goal. On the other hand, excellent work means the best work you can produce at the time with the knowledge and resources at your disposal.

When you define excellence this way, you realize it's always within reach and it should be our goal. Always!

Here's an example: Apple didn't start out by releasing iPhone 13. They could've said before the release of the first iPhone, "We should wait. It's not perfect, and with more time we could develop more features that will please our customers even more."

Instead, they released the best product they could at the time. The marketplace went wild, even though customers had a wish list for more features and functions. Apple took the feedback from the customers and created new versions every single year and in recent times, twice a year. The phones got so sophisticated that there are many award-winning movies that have been shot using the iPhone. Even with that accomplishment, they are still chasing after perfection as they continue to release new versions.

The innovations and successes of the iPhones were fantastic and historic, and they happened by focusing on excellence, not perfection. If they would've waited for perfection, they never would've released any phone, because perfection is not a realistic business strategy.

My own lesson in this came from launching my podcast. Before I started it, I had been investing time making YouTube videos regularly, and I sent out a survey about how my audience preferred to consume content. Ninety-seven percent said podcasts. Ninety-seven percent! That told me that a podcast would be an ideal way to reach and communicate with my audience.

The only problem was I barely listened to podcasts at the time myself and I surely didn't know anything about creating a podcast. If I'd let fear of failure or perfectionism have their way, I could have told myself my podcast would be lousy and would fail.

Instead, I did some basic online research about how to start a podcast and talked to my coach. This is how quickly it all came together:

- November 7: I polled my audience and found out they preferred podcasts.

- November 9: I made the decision to start a podcast and chose a platform, Buzzsprout.

- November 10: Recorded the intro and outro.

- November 12: Recorded the first three episodes.

- November 15: The podcast went live on iTunes.

- December 2: My official launch day

- December 12: We hit the one thousand downloads milestone.

In a little over a month, I went from no podcast to more than a thousand downloads.

I didn't have a fancy mic; I used the earbuds that came with my iPhone and headed to the basement, which was my "studio." I also didn't know any editors so my brother, who is a musician, had the task of editing my first episodes and adding the background music.

Eighteen months later, the podcast I launched with my iPhone and earbuds had more than one hundred thousand downloads. Was my podcast perfect? No. I just wanted to shoot for excellence and keep improving it. If there were some failures along the way, that is just part of the process on the way to success.

I should mention one more thing about the fear of failure from a business perspective. A little of it in the background can be okay. It can give you some extra motivation and edge. The key is to not let it take over or create "analysis-paralysis." Let fear sit beside you and tell it, "Watch me do what I need to do to succeed."

THE HIDDEN FEAR
YOU DIDN'T SEE COMING

Early on in my coaching, I discovered something puzzling with some of my clients.

I had some clients who showed very few fears of failure. They jumped in with both feet, built audiences of raving fans, and weren't afraid of talking in front of people—basically, everything was going great. People wanted to work with them.

But then something interesting would happen. Their prospective clients would want to book a time with them, and they never could find open spots on their calendar. Or they had a chance to close a deal on the spot, but instead they would say, "Let me get back to you."

Everything was right there, yet somehow not much was getting across the finish line, and the profits weren't happening. It didn't make any sense to me.

These were smart and capable people, and they executed well until the moment of truth. I kept digging to discover the underlying issue. To my shock, it was fear of success.

As I listened to these clients, the fear started to make more sense. They were worried that success might change them, and not for the better. They wondered, "If I become super successful, will I still have time for my family? Will I sacrifice other things that are important to me?"

Some also felt that some businesspeople have a fake veneer and that, underneath, it's all about greed and money. They wondered, "Is that who I'll become?"

If you fear success, you have the wrong idea about it. Success is like money: it's not good or bad in itself. It takes the shape of whomever has it.

If an evil person is successful, then that success will take the shape of a lot of pain and misery added to the world. If you are truly helping people, then your success will take that shape and you will add value and happiness to the world.

The beautiful thing is that I don't worry about this when it comes to my clients. Doctors are compassionate people. You didn't go into medicine with making money as your primary driver. There are a lot faster and easier ways to make money that don't take ten years of training and multiple six-figure debt.

I already know that the business you want to succeed at will add value and happiness. For example, if you succeed at a private practice, people get the care they need and you can hire staff and they can have stable jobs. Even the general community benefits from the taxes you pay.

For me, I want to succeed so tens of thousands of doctors can find financial freedom and practice medicine on their own terms. The more successful I am, the more positive the impact in the lives of others.

Another example is from a student of the EntreMD Business School. Dr. Shenelle Wilson is a fellowship-trained urologist who has started a nonprofit to help bring diversity to the field of urology. She noticed that of all the urologists in the United States, only 2 percent are Black and only 3.9 percent are Latinas. Her mission is to bring diversity into the field so that people who have urological conditions can see people who are like them and doctors who understand them culturally. If she succeeds, the whole field of urology improves. Also the patient experience for people of color will improve dramatically.

If you're fearing that success will transform you into a bad person, remember that success is not moral or immoral. It's amoral, and it takes the shape of whomever has success. It will not change you, it will simply amplify who you already are. In my experience, the world becomes a better place when we succeed.

We've conquered a fear of failure, perfectionism, and a fear of success. There's one more mindset we need to clear out of the way before we can start implementing new habits.

CHAPTER 5

Mindset Myth #3: Selling Is Not Professional

In 2009, my husband and I agreed we needed to buy a bigger car to accommodate our growing family.

I was apprehensive about going to a car dealership because of high-pressure sales tactics I'd experienced in previous car-buying adventures. My husband doesn't let that kind of thing bother him, so he was good to have along.

On our first trip out, we were immediately approached by a salesman.

"Has anybody helped you?"

We told him no, and he asked what kind of car we were looking for. We explained that we needed something with more seating, like a minivan or SUV. He immediately ushered us over to a van and launched into a monologue about why this was the best vehicle and why we needed to buy it.

He assured us the price was terrific, but the sale was going to end that day. He then wanted to hustle us off to see his manager so we could get this deal before it was too late. We explained that we wanted to go to a few more car dealerships so we could have other choices. Could we have his business card so we could revisit him if we decided we liked this van the best?

"No, I don't give people my business cards."

Was he *actually* refusing to give us his card? Yes, he was.

"When customers don't buy now, they're not going to buy later," was how he justified it to us.

Okaaayyy, then. I guess we won't be back in touch.

It's more than a decade since I had that experience, and I can still clearly recall the image of him refusing us his card.

When I thought about selling in my earlier years as an

entrepreneur, it was things like this that would come to mind. It made me hate the idea of marketing and selling. It seemed sleazy, slimy, manipulative, and selfish.

I was a professional with a heart to help people, so I told myself there was no chance I would be doing that. It took me a few years before I finally realized that selling itself is not bad. What I had experienced was bad selling, and it didn't have to be that way.

Over the years, I've thought back to that day and analyzed why it was bad selling. What was the underlying reason? It's because that salesman had no interest in creating a win for us. I wouldn't have begrudged him a win for himself, of course. If he provides a good service, why shouldn't he be rewarded? But the problem is that for him it was a one-way street. He did ask us at the very beginning what kind of vehicle we wanted, but after that it was all about pushing us into the minivan that worked best for him to sell.

He also wasn't concerned about whether it would be a win for us to make the decision on a timetable that worked for us. Instead, his win had to be today, and if that didn't work for us, that was too bad.

His every action screamed that he was just after a commission—a win for himself, and as fast as possible.

A few years later, we were once again car shopping and had a completely different experience, one that showed what good selling looks like.

This was at a luxury car dealership. The experience started the same way, with someone approaching us and asking if they could help us and what kind of car we were looking for.

As it happened, we were looking for a larger car again, an SUV. This time, the salesperson followed up with more questions. How big a family will be in the car? What will you be using it for usually—for commuting to work or for longer trips, or both? We were asked about features we might like. Everything was geared toward exploring what would make us leave with an SUV we loved and would give us value.

Next, they showed us options. Which one got better gas mileage. Which one came with better climate control. There wasn't a hint of pushing us to one choice or another. Instead, they were making every effort to find out what would make it a win for us.

Now of course, they wanted a win, too. And why not? We understood we were at a luxury dealership and weren't bargain hunting. We certainly didn't expect to overpay, but we also were willing to pay a fair price. They earned our business by making it a win for us, too. We drove away in a new SUV, with no pressure and no feeling of being "sold."

DOCTORS AND SELLING

Many doctors are excited about the idea of entrepreneurship but hate the idea of selling. They fear selling will taint them as doctors, making them appear unprofessional.

I know where they're coming from. For a time, I had the image of sales as a bit slimy, something exactly like the first car salesman who was chasing his commission without regard for who he was selling to.

Then I started making the distinction between good selling and bad selling, and it became clear to me that selling wasn't the problem. The problem was bad selling.

Doctors are right to not engage in bad selling, but we should become masters of good selling. Why? Because selling is a vehicle that creates wins for everyone. If you stop to think about it, I bet you can come up with several problems in your life right now that you would happily pay someone to solve.

If someone walks up to you with the solution, you win because your problem goes away and the person wins because she got paid (rewarded) for serving you. This leads me to the conclusion that while bad selling is bad, good selling is great!

Your attitude towards selling will change when you understand that not telling people about your product or service blocks their access to a better life.

A great example of this is Dr. Michelle Quirk, a student in the EntreMD Business School. Her story is very interesting, and we'll return to it again later in the book, but here's a quick version to help us understand why selling the right way is good.

Michelle is now a running coach, but you wouldn't have guessed that if you had known her earlier in life. She became a runner relatively late. She lacked confidence in her running ability to the point that at first she didn't think she could run a 5K. But of course she could, and she did eventually.

Next, she didn't think she could become a marathoner, but she conquered that, too.

Running became a passion of hers with outstanding benefits. She felt healthier, her mood was better, and she had the overwhelming sense of accomplishment that spilled over to other aspects of her life.

She realized she could start a business as a run coach and teach others the skills and help them develop the confidence to create the same transformation. She became certified and went on to coach many others to accomplish their own first 5Ks, 10Ks, half marathons, and full marathons. In many cases, it has transformed the lives of her clients. How does she know that it changes their lives? They tell her.

She hears things like: "I'm forty-three years old and I always secretly wanted to do a marathon. But at my age, I figured it was too late to start and that I never would accomplish it. Now I completed my first marathon and it's been life changing. That I could reach that milestone is one of the highlights of my life."

Dr. Quirk has discovered there are many, many people out there with this unlived part of themselves, and she's in a unique position to help them find a way to a new, more fulfilled life. They have a dream, and she has the solution.

If she stayed stuck in a fear of selling her coaching services, would her clients ever find a way to their running dreams? The truth is most of them wouldn't. That's not just a loss of business for Dr. Quirk; it would be sad for all the people who would never reach their goals.

Here's another great example. I had the pleasure of interviewing a radiation oncologist and physician entrepreneur, Dr. Katie Deming. She has a completely different story that makes essentially the same point. She witnessed firsthand that there was a need for a more comfortable bra for breast cancer patients who had undergone radiation therapy. Normal bras cause increased pain and irritation after treatment, so she came up with an idea for a bra that was much more comfortable.

She went on to create a very successful company called Makemerry. This wonderful idea that she came up with has given comfort to thousands of people at a time when they really need it.

These two very different businesses are absolutely life changing for the people who need them.

The question we need to ask is this: what would have happened to all the people who were helped by this running coach or by a more comfortable bra if either of these business owners had said, "I don't want to sell. I'm afraid it will make me look unprofessional and that I only care about money"?

The simple truth is that all the benefits their clients and customers received never would've happened. The dreams of many would-be runners would've stayed unfulfilled wishes. The extra years those runners added to their lives through better fitness would disappear. The relief felt by those breast cancer patients who did not have to suffer with the wrong bra would never have happened.

When you grasp this insight, you see that a refusal to sell is not neutral. It's actually a disservice. I find the fear of selling understandable, but I also get a little frustrated with it. If what you offer has value to people, why would you not want to sell it to them?

Help people have better lives. Tell them how your product or service can do that. When you don't, you're blocking them from a better life.

SOMEONE HAS BEEN SELLING FOR YOU

As I've mentioned previously, when I started a private practice in 2010, I got a quick dose of reality. Patients weren't going to be banging down my door just because I opened a practice. It would take business skills, especially sales and marketing, to make the practice viable.

How did I not realize that? I think I'm like many doctors who were somewhat insulated from the business side of medicine.

Let's say you're a doctor working in an outpatient clinic or in a hospital-owned practice. You report to work, grab a cup of coffee, chat with a few coworkers, and then dive into your day seeing patients. The patients are already on the schedule, so you just see them. At the end of the pay period, you get paid. All of this can create a little bit of an illusion that patients just find us without any sales or marketing, and that the paychecks will always keep coming.

But the truth is that clinics, hospitals, and privately owned practices are all doing sales and marketing to fill up that schedule. People have to know where to go for a solution to their medical issue, and also why they should choose a particular facility or practice.

Patients don't show up by magic, but when you aren't involved on the business side of medicine, it can be easy to be a bit naive about that. When you think about selling as unprofessional or "undoctorly," remember that someone is likely doing it on your behalf, and it's how you stay employed.

This is why we think that if we just open a practice, people will come. Or if we have a great product or service, there's no need to sell it—people will find it and love it. But it doesn't work that way.

MAKE THE CONNECTION BETWEEN SALES AND SOLUTIONS

The best cure for thinking of sales as something unprofessional or sleazy is to understand that you are providing a solution to people, as we saw in the examples above.

If you struggle with ridding yourself of the mindset of sales as something bad, affirm these three things:

• What I offer has value.

• People are looking for what I offer.

• People are willing to pay for what I offer.

Let's look at an example of how this might work. Let's say you're offering a program to help people overcome obesity. Many people who sign up and pay for your program are losing weight, learning how to eat better, and even exercising for the first time in their lives.

Most of the people in the program also have others in the family who are overweight, plus have all the hypertension, diabetes, and heart trouble that come with it. By participating in your program, they're demonstrating a whole new paradigm for their entire family.

Next, maybe some medications become unnecessary, and the client starts to perform with more energy and focus at work—everything is changing. You're changing a life dramatically.

Will people value an offer to reduce obesity and feel more in control of their lives? Are people looking for a way to rid themselves of obesity? Are people willing to pay for solutions to obesity? The answer is a resounding yes to all three.

You should also notice that when it comes to obesity solutions, there are others in the marketplace willing to sell things that don't work. Isn't it better that you are out there actively selling a solution grounded in science and medically sound advice?

If you're unwilling to promote your solution, how many lives will not be transformed? If you take the time to think about it, the numbers will shock you.

Here's an example from my business. There are one million physicians in the United States. Even if only 10 percent need my help, that's one hundred thousand physicians. Potentially there are one hundred thousand physicians who want to start or scale businesses but can't figure out how. If I truly have the answer that can help them, it's wrong to shy away from selling.

The best way to bust the "selling is unprofessional" myth is to sit down and really reflect on the value you're offering, then reframe it as solutions you're bringing to people who need it. Once you do this, it's time to sell.

PART THREE

REENGINEER YOUR ACTIONS

CHAPTER 6

Getting Your Daily Habits Right

What ultimately determines your success? Is it pretty much just a combination of circumstances, inborn talent, and luck? Author and leadership expert John Maxwell doesn't think so:

> If I could come to your house and spend just one day with you, I would be able to tell whether or not you will be successful. You could pick the day. If I got up with you in the morning and went through the day with you, watching you for twenty-four hours, I could tell in what direction your life is headed.

Maxwell also provides the answer to what you *should* be doing every day: a routine of constructive habits. "You'll never change your life until you change something you do daily. The secret of your success is found in your daily routine."

As we move from mindsets to the chapters on habits and actions, the first thing to understand is the importance of daily habits. They will form the foundation of everything else. You need new habits to help reinforce your new mindsets.

I remember reading those thoughts from John Maxwell years ago and having them instantly resonate with me. Even so, I didn't understand just how transformative daily habits could be until I implemented them.

Understanding that daily habits are the difference between success and failure brings an accountability to our lives. We can no longer live in the world of self-deception, where outward circumstances, other people, or luck determine our fate. We have to accept that in most cases, we are the bottleneck in our lives, blocking ourselves from progress.

Circumstances and luck may have their say in the short run, but in the long run our success rests with us and what we do on a daily basis. Soon after reading the Maxwell quote, I happened to be watching a YouTube video created by Terri Savelle Foy, where she talked about her own routine.

What struck me was how simple it was. It helped me realize that there was no need to waste heaps of time coming up with some elaborate plan for the perfect daily routine. She did five simple things every day: pray, meditate, read, exercise, and listen to a motivational message.

I decided I could choose equally simple things and focus on doing them every day.

It changed everything.

THE NINE CORE AREAS OF LIFE

I teach that there are nine core areas of life:

- Family

- Health

- Career/Business

- Intellectual Development

- Fun

- Social Capital

- Spirituality

- Legacy

Now you might be wondering why I would include this list of core areas of life in a business book. The answer is that they are fundamental, and your daily habits should help you make progress in these essential areas.

When key areas of our life are misfiring, it's going to impact our ability to be present in our business. It causes us to bring less to our work that we are capable of. The flip side is also true. The better these areas are functioning, the more energy and positivity we'll bring to our entrepreneurial efforts.

I've come up with six daily habits that help me stay connected and moving forward in these nine core areas of life.

Prayer/Meditation

My relationship with God is very important. I know when I make this a priority every day, it will ensure that the relationship strengthens. This habit creates an oasis of calm and peace and helps me consistently dream big dreams. Every day, I take the time to pray and meditate on the scriptures.

Exercise

I do this for a very simple reason. Ignoring your health can rob you of years of your life. Poor physical health also means you won't be able to show up to the other areas of your life with the energy and focus those areas deserve. This habit does not need to be overwhelming. When I started, all I did was a thirty-minute walk. Remember that doing a little consistently is so much more powerful than doing a lot once in a while.

Listen to Podcasts

This is part of my intellectual development, which is very important to me. I attentively search for a valuable nugget to take away from every podcast I listen to. This adds to my store of business knowledge and general life wisdom.

Read

I also do this for intellectual development. Setting aside thirty minutes of your day for a business book, personal development, or spiritual topic will spur tremendous growth over time.

Review My Goals

I make a point of reviewing my goals every day. It's how I stay on track.

This is something I began doing after an eye-opening experience I had in December 2015. I sat down to write out my goals for 2016. After I was done, I happened to glance at my goals for 2015 and was shocked to see my goals were identical.

Somehow, I had let myself live on autopilot for an entire year. I had written down goals, but I had failed to check in on them. I had been "busy" all year, but I had stopped moving forward because I didn't keep my goals front and center. So now I make sure I check in with them daily.

MTWK

My other daily habit I call MTWK, which is an acronym that stands for Meaningful Time With Kids. It reminds me that every day I need to spend quality time with my kids.

As many doctors are, I'm a type A personality. That can be good for business and career and other goals, but focused personalities can sometimes have trouble slowing down and being present with kids, spouses, and friends.

On top of that, we live in weird times where a family can sit in the same room but be in their own separate worlds of individual devices. To have meaningful exchanges, we need to commit to them.

One of the things I love about daily habits is that I can't have a day where I don't make progress in the core areas of life. I could have a day where everything else goes wrong and feels like a complete failure on the surface, but I still know that some good did happen and I made significant progress because of my daily routine.

STEAL THIS ROUTINE

If you're not sure where to start your own daily routine, you can begin with mine. You'll eventually tweak or maybe even significantly change it, but for now, it's much more important to get started than to worry about designing a perfect routine.

The power of "stealing" a proven routine hit home for me based on the experience of a friend. She was going through a rough patch and was really struggling. Trying to pull herself out of her funk by herself wasn't working. In the frame of mind she was in, designing her own daily habits wasn't an option either.

So I told her I didn't want her to be anxious about creating her own routine, I simply wanted her to borrow mine. I heard from her again four weeks later.

"I don't understand exactly how or why it worked, but you changed my life."

Her results in just four weeks were dramatic. Her mood was transformed and her previous feelings of burnout at work were gone. In fact, she was making more money than she had previously because of increased productivity. She'd also lost weight and put an offer in on a new home, something she had procrastinated on for years. When you change what you do every day, everything can change for you.

I strongly recommend not overthinking this. Get started now and edit the routine later!

FINDING TIME

One of the most common objections I hear from clients is, "I won't be able to find the time."

I have some sympathy for this sentiment, but whenever I hear it, I think back to 2010.

At the time, I was working twenty hours a week at the local urgent care to take care of bills while also building my new practice. I had a two-year-old and a four-month-old. My weekends were not free, either, because my husband and I pastor a church. I still found time for daily habits.

To be sure, I had to be creative about it. I would pray and meditate immediately after waking up. I would pace back and forth while I did that so I could get at least two thousand steps in on my fitness tracker.

Then I would find a podcast to listen to and let it play while I took a shower and got ready for work. My goals were in my journal so I would look at them and read them back to myself as though they had already happened. After that, it was time to get into the car and drive to work, and I would listen to an audiobook on my commute. After work, it would be time for MTWK.

When I hear time complaints from my clients, I ask them some questions: Can you take a fifteen-minute walk every day? Or listen to an audiobook in the car on your way to work for thirty minutes? Can you open your eyes in the morning and start praying or meditating?

Still, I do understand the time pressures all of us are under. That's exactly why we want to keep our daily habits simple but powerful. You'll find the time if you want to do this.

MORE THOUGHTS ON
A DAILY ROUTINE OF HABITS

I want to leave you with some helpful tips and reflections on instituting daily habits in your own life. It's a crucial step in your journey, so please heed anything that can help you implement these changes.

- Watch for the compound effect of daily habits. It's definitely like investing money wisely: as time goes by, your returns start earning interest. Habits create the same impact when you do them every day.

- Don't fall into the trap of focusing on slipups. I have some clients who immediately feel doomed if they miss a day after a good streak of days. Instead of obsessing about a missed day, acknowledge that you're human and then immediately pour your energy into getting right back into your routine the next day. Anything else is self-sabotage.

- Don't expect instant results. In fact, don't expect results at all, because that can start to block you and create anxiety. Results happen when we stay focused on the intention and execution of your daily habits. Let the rewards follow naturally without fixating on them.

- Notice when you start seeing benefits in other areas of your life not directly related to your daily habits. This happens because how you do one thing is how you do everything. The consistency of daily habits will bleed over into other actions, and you'll be amazed by the impact.

Most of all, I want you to start doing this. It's the execution of the simple things that changes lives. You can finish reading this chapter and think, "That is so interesting," and then never do anything about it.

Or you can get going now and watch it radically transform your life. That's why I suggest you use my routine, at least for now. It's the perfect way to get started without over-thinking it.

Getting your daily habits in line is the foundation of all your other actions. And then it'll be time to stretch yourself beyond your normal boundaries.

CHAPTER 7

Get Comfortable Being Uncomfortable

In Chapter 5, I introduced one of my EntreMD Business School students, Dr. Michelle Quirk, when we talked about overcoming the fear of failure and the fear of selling.

That's a crucial mindset change, but what actions did it lead to for her? And what results did she get?

I used to joke with Michelle that her business as a running coach was the world's best-kept secret. Michelle, despite being an introvert, eventually decided it shouldn't be a secret anymore and went out and lived outside her comfort zone.

In a twelve-month period of time, these were some of her accomplishments:

- Went from a small handful of videos on her YouTube channel to over forty-two videos, including a series of conversations with runners and thought leaders in her field.

- Did twenty guest podcast interviews after only doing five the entire previous year.

- Almost quadrupled her email list, from around eighty to over three hundred.

- Hosted one workshop and was a guest in two virtual summits.

- Got multiple paid speaking gigs including guest coaching opportunities and women's conferences.

- Started to grow her team, including a virtual assistant to help with social media and two college interns to help with blog writing.

- Hosted her first virtual 5K.

- Not only did her clients achieve many running milestones, they also lost hundreds of pounds.

- In addition to all this, she was able to negotiate and cut her clinical time to three days per week starting January 2022!

For her business, the results of all this action were amazing. By September 2021, she had already surpassed three times what she made in all of 2020. That demonstrates the power of putting yourself out there. She did all of this while working full time as a pediatrician.

Michelle realized that if she was going to thrive as an entrepreneur, she had to redefine the word *uncomfortable*.

No matter who we are, almost all of us prefer to stay in a comfort zone. It's completely human to want to stick with things we know and are good at. Feeling competent and in control gives our emotions a boost, while leaving that zone makes us feel unsure of ourselves.

If you want to be successful as an entrepreneur, you're going to need to take consistent action outside your comfort zone. If you do this long enough, you can actually get to the point where you become comfortable being uncomfortable. I like to inspire my students by telling them that my permanent address is now, "PO Box: Outside My Comfort Zone." This is where all the growth happens.

That may sound impossible to you if you're naturally shy, but if introverts like myself and Michelle can do it, you can follow the same path.

I want to point out that this chapter is where you take all the previous mindsets that you're trying to change and make them real in the world of action. You'll put aside fear of failure and anxieties about selling. You'll stop listening to the voice that says, "I'm just a doctor."

The magical thing is that when you take action in the face of these mindsets, it reinforces your new mindsets and changes your business. As you see real results (like Michelle did when her revenue rose dramatically in 2021), your confidence soars and you become willing to get outside your comfort zone more and more.

As an entrepreneur, life-changing results will always be found outside your circle of comfort. You've got to retrain yourself. When you start to feel uncomfortable, that's not an invitation to stop. It's a reliable indication that you've just bumped up against the boundary of your comfort zone, and a sure sign you need to keep going.

Eventually, you will feel excitement when you bump up against discomfort, and be thrilled to face a challenge—even though the fear or discomfort won't completely disappear.

DO TALK TO STRANGERS

You probably heard the message "don't talk to strangers" a lot as a child. We were given books with safety themes that included this message. It was embedded in television programs, and of course our parents reinforced this message. It's an appropriate message for young people to keep them from strangers who may mean them harm.

For many of us, however, it stays our default as adults, even after it no longer serves us well. It's an especially bad idea for entrepreneurs.

According to Brian Tracy, the author of *Eat That Frog* whom we met in Chapter 3, typically about 80 percent of the people who would love your products or services—and would happily pay for them—have no idea you exist.

It won't matter at all if you have a valuable product or service that solves a problem if the people who have that problem have never heard of you.

Your job is the exact opposite of what was ingrained into you as a kid. You must talk to strangers. You need to seek out audiences—both online and in person—and talk to them. The more strangers you talk to, the more successful your business will be.

PROMOTING YOURSELF

When you hear the words "promote yourself," what comes to mind? For too many doctors, they imagine this as going out in the world to puff themselves up. But promoting yourself isn't about saying, "Look how great I am."

Our training as physicians often works against the idea of promoting ourselves. This is related to the anxieties about selling that we talked about previously. Many doctors who work inside a practice, or hospital, or clinic don't see that someone is doing the promoting for them. The marketing is still happening, we're just not making the connection.

Remember that promoting yourself is really about getting your solution (product or service or both) to people who need that solution. It's mandatory for success.

Unfortunately, understanding in your head that you are helping people find a solution doesn't completely erase the discomfort. No doubt, Michelle felt strange hosting her first virtual summit. As entrepreneurs, we all have that feeling sometimes of "Who am I to do this?"

When you put yourself out there—creating videos, going to networking events, introducing yourself to strangers, being a guest or a host of a podcast—you'll feel deeply uncomfortable at times, and sometimes just...well, weird. But when you remind yourself that it's a normal and expected part of the process, you can push through it.

"I DIDN'T DIE"

How much do we all fear being outside our comfort zone?

A common theme in comments from the EntreMD Business School students is a good indication:

- *"I did my first video and I didn't die!"*

- *"I went on that TV segment and I'm still alive!"*

- *"My first podcast is up on iTunes and it didn't actually kill me!"*

Of course, no one expects to actually die from promoting their business, but it's revealing that "I didn't die" is how people gently poke fun at how deep their fears can be around promoting themselves and their businesses. You are not alone.

BUT WHAT IF I STILL FEEL ALONE?

It's all well and good for me to tell you that promoting yourself is mandatory and nothing to be timid about. And it probably provides some comfort to understand that you're not alone in your fears.

But what do you do if understanding this in your head isn't enough? What do you do when you need help actually crossing that boundary and heading into discomfort's zip code?

Coaching and community is the answer.

I'm betting if you were given an option to skip doing a spinal tap during your residency training, you never would've done one. I know I probably wouldn't have had the courage to do that without it being required. When it's mandatory, you find a way to do it. There's no putting it off.

This is why I love coaching and community. It keeps us accountable and forces us to move forward. If you're in a community of like-minded doctors who are all embracing discomfort, then it becomes normalized, a kind of positive peer pressure.

But the benefits go well beyond pushing you past fear. It's also the encouragement and positive feedback you get when you do go outside your comfort zone. It's about sharing ideas on what promotion efforts are working, or sometimes coming together to create content together, giving you strength in numbers.

RID YOURSELF OF THE IDEA THAT YOUR PRODUCT OR SERVICE WILL "SELL ITSELF"

No matter the evidence, some doctors have trouble shaking the idea that an excellent product or service should be enough by itself to be successful. They think that if you put all your efforts into building it, people will see it and they will find you.

In movieland, when you build it, they will come. But in real life, they don't. The saying of podcaster and entrepreneur John Lee Dumas is more accurate: "If you build it, they will not care until you make them aware."

Many new entrepreneurs will spend 90 to 100 percent of their time building their product or service, fiddling with a new website, and coming up with the perfect colors for their logo. Seasoned entrepreneurs realize that the split between developing your product or service and promoting it has to be much closer to a fifty-fifty time investment. You need to spend at least as much time telling people about your solution as you do developing it.

Don't spend all your time building the perfect baseball diamond in a cornfield. Or in our case, building some beautiful product or service that will serve people, but then leave it hidden on a website nobody visits. As doctors, we want our product or service to be perfect first. But just like the first iPhone, we need to shoot for excellence, then release it and tell as many people as we can.

I mentioned John Lee Dumas above, and he's an instructive example. He wrote a terrific book called *The Common Path to Uncommon Success*. To promote that book, he did 345 interviews *in less than three months*. John also reached out to 3,010 individuals to ask for their support on the launch! He no doubt spent a lot of time making his book excellent, but he did not assume that meant people would find it. He made as many people aware as possible.

What makes this even more fascinating is the fact that he has a podcast with over one million downloads a month. He could have easily made the assumption that he didn't need to do any promotion other than mentioning his book on his podcast. But he knew it would take more than that. No wonder he ended up with a very successful book launch and 533 reviews on Amazon.

Another great example is Michelle Obama, one of the most famous women in America. As a former first lady, if anybody could say, "I'll write a good book, and people will find it," it's her. But she supported the launch with a national book tour to thirty-three cities. Yes, it probably would've been a bestseller regardless, but it's now one of the best-selling memoirs of all time. It sold more than two million copies in fifteen days.

You have to make people aware if you want extraordinary results.

There's a catch to all this, however. As you put yourself outside your comfort zone, you may discover that you have some skill gaps you need to close.

CHAPTER 8

The Power of Personal Development

By 2017, I had been running my practice for seven years, everything was going great, and there was nothing to complain about. But I couldn't shake the nagging feeling that something was missing. I wanted more.

The only problem was I didn't know what I meant by "more" or how I might go about finding it.

Around that time, I spotted a small ad for a three-day speakers boot camp. I thought to myself, "I would love to be able to be a more confident speaker and not be terrified of the stage."

Of course, right on cue, a bunch of negative thoughts flooded my brain, immediately going to war with this idea.

"You're the very definition of an introvert. That's who you are. You'll be petrified the entire time."

I decided to go anyway. And, truth be told, I was terrified at least some of the time. We had to do some practice exercises during the weekend, including a three-minute talk that scared me spitless.

But there was a flip side. I was absolutely exhilarated by what I was discovering. Speaking was a skill you could learn, and it didn't matter whether you were an introvert or an extrovert. The boot camp provided frameworks for speaking that transformed my perspective.

On day two, the event organizers talked about a ten-month speaking mastermind program that we were invited to join. As I saw what I could learn in the program, I was excited and started thinking that maybe this was something I should do.

And then they talked about the investment: $43,000.

FORTY. THREE. THOUSAND. DOLLARS.

My first thought: "They're insane."

And my second thought was the same: "No, really, are they crazy? $43,000 for ten months? To be a better speaker?" I was feeling borderline indignant about their audacity.

But after the initial shock, my thinking began evolving in another direction. Hadn't I already seen excellent results in two days? Wouldn't being able to speak more confidently be a game-changer for my business and my life? What would that be worth?

I began focusing less on the cost and instead started looking at the program through the lens of value. Of course, that still didn't mean I made a snap decision. I took some more time to consider the details of the program. I thought more about how they had already proved their expertise to me during the boot camp. I talked it over with my husband. And in the end, I decided to invest in my personal development, even if the price tag made me want to faint.

That decision would change my life. How much it transformed my skills really hit home for me after speaking in 2021 at our annual event called EntreMD Live. Over five hundred doctors registered for our event that year, and I received so much generous and amazing feedback.

"Your message was so clear." "Your talk was so inspirational." "You gave us clear action steps." But there was another piece of feedback I heard several times that had me chuckling to myself:

"You're such a natural speaker."

I, of course, thanked everyone who called me a natural, but I couldn't help but smile and think, "I'm the furthest thing from a natural speaker you'll ever meet!"

To this day, I still consider myself an introverted introvert. It's just that I invested in learning professional-level speaking skills and practiced them. There was absolutely nothing natural about it. Looking back, that $43,000 investment has paid for itself many times over because of how it's helped EntreMD grow. It's made this super-shy, socially awkward introvert into someone who can speak on stage in front of hundreds of physicians multiple times a year and create over four hundred YouTube videos. It's allowed me to create a podcast with more than one hundred thousand downloads in ninety-one countries in eighteen months.

My husband always refers to it as the best $43,000 we ever spent.

WHERE DO YOU INVEST THE MOST?

You need to think of yourself as the asset with the ability to appreciate more than anything else in your life.

Say you decide to invest to remodel your kitchen at a cost of $40,000. That will increase the value of your home. But is it maybe a higher priority to invest in ourselves and our businesses? When we invest in ourselves strategically, we can earn it back many times over, and then maybe build a $100,000 kitchen.

It's crucial that you understand that YOU are and will always be the most important asset in your business. Your business can't grow faster than your skills allow. I sometimes hear someone say, "I'm going to have a big year." I love the enthusiasm, but based on what? You'll have that big year when you invest in yourself to increase your skills, not just by saying it. Investment in yourself is always mandatory (a lesson you already learned by investing yourself in becoming a doctor).

The more time you can spend in personal development, the faster progress you'll make.

ENROLL IN
AUTOMOBILE UNIVERSITY

One of the simplest ways to develop more skills is also one of the best: turning your commute time into a continuing education. I learned this concept from Terri Savelle Foy many years ago and when she referred to it as "Automobile University." It means finding audio courses, podcasts, and audiobooks that address the skills you need to learn and invest your time in the car in consuming those materials.

It needs to be emphasized that you need to be strategic about what you choose. For example, when I first opened my practice, hiring the right people was a big problem for me. Staffing became a revolving-door situation with too much turnover. But remembering that all business skills are learnable, I went in search of something that could teach me hiring skills and how to build a great company culture.

I purchased a Brian Tracy audio program on how to hire and fire. This meant my commute time was strategically focused on the exact weakness I had. Your time is not unlimited; don't just listen to anything. It's tempting to listen to anything that's good, but it's still a poor choice if it's not addressing a deep need of yours.

Of course, I'm not saying general motivation isn't great, too. I feed myself a steady diet of inspiring content, because I find inspiration wears off quickly otherwise. I especially seek out autobiographies of leaders, entrepreneurs, and influential figures from public life for that purpose. When I read about some of the challenges that people overcome, it's breathtaking.

If these leaders could overcome their mountains, how could I even think about quitting because of the hills in front of me? It also reminds me on tough days not to get thrown off balance. Every time I listen to an autobiography or a podcast about an entrepreneurial journey, it always ends up helping me show up better in my own life and business.

Here are some more tips for getting the most out of Automobile University:

- If your commute is too short, or you work from home, don't overlook the options to listen during a walk, when getting ready for your day, or while doing mindless chores. (I call this "Downtime University," where you use what would otherwise be mundane task time to improve yourself.)

- Wherever you listen, it's good to make this a "set it and forget it" thing. You want to be able to turn the ignition on your car, press play, and go. If it's a valued podcast, get the alert that tells you when a new one drops and click it the next time you're in the car. The more automatic, the better.

- Some of my clients say they need their car time as downtime to relax from the other rigorous parts of their day. My recommendation to them is to split the commute time. Use the commute to work when you are fresh for Automobile University and then use the commute home for calling a friend or listening to happy music.

LEADERS ARE READERS

As much as I benefit from being able to learn with audio so as not to waste time in the car, it shouldn't be viewed as a complete replacement for reading books.

The plain fact is that leaders are readers. That's an inescapable conclusion. Bill Gates is worth billions, coleads a huge foundation, and still reads fifty books a year. Mark Cuban has 150 companies, is worth $4.5 billion, and he makes time to read three hours a day.

Physical books are worth spending time with because it's much harder to get distracted. If you're reading on a tablet, there's a lot of potential for alerts popping up, or the temptation to click on a link in the text. With an audiobook, you can be listening and then realize you drifted off for five minutes and suddenly snap back thinking, "What's being talked about?"

Reading physical books is one of the best resources for

personal development, but I also don't want to fall into the trap of those who try to motivate people to read using guilt tactics. Saying things like, "You should be reading a book a week or you're doing it wrong" isn't helpful.

Instead of hectoring yourself about not reading enough, try this: aim to read more than you do currently. If you're at zero books a month, start reading one book a month. That should be your absolute minimum. If you're already doing a book a month, see if you can go to two books a month, and so on.

One last piece of advice on reading: don't choose books based on titles; choose based on authors. I always look at the author's credentials and track record. Before I spend my valuable time, I need to know they've "been there, done that," because they can't give what they don't have.

If you're writing about business success and haven't had any, I'm not selecting your book, no matter how catchy your title is.

TAKE THE SHORTCUT TO SUCCESS

It's commonly claimed, "There's no shortcut to success." Wrong.

For everything you're trying to do in business, someone has been there before. They've already done it. They've gone to the school of hard knocks, made the mistakes, and learned the lessons. With the right coaching or community, you can shave years off your learning curve.

Of course, a shortcut doesn't mean you won't have to work hard. It won't eliminate all your mistakes. But to say that mentors, coaches, and programs can't accelerate your personal development and your skills acquisition is simply false. I know because people have helped me "collapse time" and get where I'm going faster, and I've helped others do the same.

Of course, that doesn't mean all mentors, coaches, programs, and communities are created equal. The best way to appraise them is to look at the free resources created by the coach or mentor. Videos, podcasts, blogs, and more are typically available.

Go there and consume the content. Take the advice for a test drive and see if you can generate wins by applying it. Get a feel for the coach's style and look carefully for evidence of results they get with their clients. And check out their own business and how they present it. These are all clues.

Please don't decide on something after clicking on an online ad and then being taken to a sales page where they imply you better buy today or your life is destined for failure. There's no emergency here.

Choosing a program should be a carefully considered executive decision, not a whim. At the same time, remember that absolute perfect information does not exist. Don't spend forever trying to make a decision. It's human nature to go to one extreme or the other. Take the time to research a program, but also don't delay endlessly. Quickly make the best decision you can with the information you gather from your research.

This is a lot like how I decided to pay $43,000 to become a better speaker. I only decided to invest after a weekend seminar had demonstrated that the leaders knew what they were talking about and could deliver great results. However, once I knew they could help me, I quickly made the decision to invest.

It's also important to remember that there are many coaches and programs that are wonderful but still the wrong decision for you. This goes back to the idea of strategically choosing resources that specifically address the skills you need to develop.

WHAT'S YOUR LEVEL OF COMMITMENT?

Having a good coach or enrolling in a great program is no guarantee of success. It's like a good marriage: it takes two to make it work. I know a lot of people who focus on whether the program or coach would give them a money-back guarantee. There is nothing wrong with that if you're truly concerned that the program might not deliver value. But many times people want a guarantee as an escape valve instead of fully committing to their own success.

There's no program on the market handing out magic beans. The formula for results is a good program plus a good participant. Anytime you pay for coaching, a program, or to join a community, make the decision to be the person who gets the most out of it.

Do whatever is within your power to attend every event and class, put your full effort into the assignments, ask lots of questions, and be fully engaged.

Believe it or not, some of my fellow students in the $43,000 program didn't do the work. I'm betting some of them would say the program didn't work and was overpriced. It sure worked for me, because I used the program to change my life. I promised myself I would be one of the best students they ever had, and my ROI has been incredible.

Even if as a physician you have a significant time crunch, you can still choose to do your best. When I did the speaking program, the majority of the assignments were to speak at events. That would require more time off work to travel to conferences than I could afford to do at the time.

My solution was to find another way to take action, so I started doing Facebook Live broadcasts every single week. I used that as my platform to practice all the concepts I was learning. When you make a firm decision to get the most out of a program, you can become creative in making it happen.

Here's an example, this time from my students. At the EntreMD Business School, we have live sessions every Wednesday. There are students who can't always show up live every week. But some of them have committed to listen to the replays on Thursday when they can't make the live session. I admire that they've made a quality decision to get the most out of the program, even when their schedule forces them to make an adjustment.

My advice: any time you pay for a personal development coaching or program, decide to be one of the best students who ever participated. Make that commitment. Remember that what you get out of it is up to you, and you have to do the work. The coach or the program is not the hero—they can help you go faster but they're not flying in with a cape to save the day. You are the hero of your story—it's like breathing; you can't delegate it.

FORGING RELATIONSHIPS

There's another shortcut I wish I'd learned earlier as an entrepreneur, and that's the transformational power of relationships. Relationships matter.

You've probably heard the saying that you are the average of the five people you spend the most time with. I think that's true, but developing relationships with mega-successful people has the potential to create radical, dramatic transformation in your life. To thrive as an entrepreneur, you have to strategically position yourself among other entrepreneurs.

The friends we have from elementary school, as neighbors, as college roommates, are friendships by default, given to us by the circumstances of life. Of course, those can be wonderful friendships and I'm not advocating neglecting those that are important to you.

But you also need to think strategically about your other relationships. Let's say you've grown to $100,000 in revenue a year. If your next goal is to leap to a half million a year, you're going to need to find people who are running half-a-million-dollar businesses and find a way to connect with that circle of people.

By entering that circle, your belief in what's possible naturally gets elevated. Spend enough time on these relationships, and a half million a year in revenue will go from a dream to your expectation. You'll also get access to the strategies that work for them. You might think they would be stingy with those strategies, but my experience with successful people is the opposite. They truly want to help others.

The insight about the power of relationships really hit home for me watching a YouTube video. The person hosting the video was running a multimillion-dollar business, and he scored a private meeting with a billionaire. He asked the billionaire what the difference was between a millionaire and a billionaire.

The answer instantly resonated with me: millionaires focus on ideas and implementation, but billionaires focus on collaboration.

You might be thinking discussing billionaires is a little advanced for the stage you're at. My take is that if billionaires focus on collaboration, then we might as well start practicing right now!

What are some ways to forge relationships with successful people?

Let me give you three ideas to start with.

First, network at events. Introverted me used to skulk in the back of event halls, listen to the speaker, and then dart for the door the second they were over. I'm still an introvert, but I've developed new skills. Now I sit right up front, and when the event is done, I walk up to the speaker and introduce myself.

I give them a genuine compliment and tell them what resonated with me. Maybe it leads to something, maybe it doesn't, but meet enough influential people and you will see results from it.

Two, if you host a podcast or YouTube channel, that's a terrific opportunity to do outreach. Who can you interview for your podcast? When you bring on successful people, your audience wins, because they hear useful stories. Sometimes it will lead to a big win for you with an ongoing relationship with the guest.

Third, community can change you. Some communities are "pay to play." If that's what it takes to make connections that will propel you forward, then pay. Relationships make the difference—by elevating your own belief of what's possible, by opening doors for you, and by teaching you strategies.

You've cleared out damaging mindsets. You've learned important ways to take action. Now it's finally time to find the right business idea for you.

PART FOUR

GETTING DOWN TO BUSINESS

CHAPTER 9

Find Your Idea

In 2017, I traveled to the UK for a big family party following my niece's graduation as an aerospace engineer. While on that trip, I got to reconnect with a friend of mine from high school, Dr. Yinka, a fellow physician.

As we talked, I was struck by her passion for skin care for women of color. It seemed like she was on a mission to help women of color reverse the aging process so they can look years younger (which, personally speaking, sounds like music to my ears!).

She explained to me that she was often told by her patients, "I'd like to get rid of some wrinkles, but I don't want to do Botox. I don't like needles."

So Dr. Yinka started experimenting with regimens of sunscreen, washes, and creams that would fight aging skin without needles. By the time I was talking to her, she was already getting terrific results for herself and others.

I was fascinated, and I couldn't help but notice that what she was telling me added up to a fantastic business idea. She had everything she needed to get started. She was passionate about the subject. She was already experimenting with skin-care regimens backed by science that were producing consistent results. And she had an audience who had clearly told her they had a problem (aging skin), but were not willing to use the conventional solutions like Botox and other procedures.

Then she confided to me, "I've been wanting to start my own skin-care line, but that's not something I can do."

I asked why she couldn't do it. She ticked off a long list of reasons why not. To my ears, not a single one held water.

I took the conversation in a different direction. When was her birthday, I asked? November 27, she told me.

"I'll work with you, and we'll get you set up to launch your own skin-care line on your birthday," I said.

She agreed to go for it. She then overcame every hurdle that year and on her fortieth birthday, she launched Dr. Yinka Skin—her own skin-care line. She had four core products that every woman of color should be using, which she called the Vital Four: sunscreen, glycolic acid wash, retinol, and vitamin C serum. Since the day she launched, I have used only her products for my skin because they are just that good.

It's stories like these that reinforce my belief that every physician has a seven-figure business idea in them.

FIVE QUESTIONS TO FIND A GREAT BUSINESS IDEA

When I first talk to doctors about launching a business, many of them have a desire for it but are unsure of how to find an idea. I use a series of five questions to help them discover the idea they already have somewhere inside them.

What problems have you solved for yourself and others?

This is one of the best ways to find a business idea. For example, this is the whole basis for EntreMD. I had made the journey from "doctor with no business skills" to a successful entrepreneur with a thriving business, which in my case was a private practice. Now I help other doctors make the same transition.

Another example I love in this category is Jamie Kern Lima. She suffered from rosacea and couldn't find makeup on the market that worked for her. So she came up with her own makeup to solve her own problem. Then she realized there were millions and millions of people out there with skin issues, and all the makeup products were geared toward people without skin problems.

She ended up launching her own makeup based on the problem she had solved for herself. She eventually sold her business to L'Oréal for $1.1 billion.

What skills/certifications do you have?

Many doctors have been trained in other areas besides treating patients, but they don't often recognize those as special skills. To them, it's just something they do that's normal.

For example, maybe you've been certified on a new electronic health record system, and you helped onboard the entire hospital. Or maybe you train students as a normal part of your duties. That takes skill. We're too often blind to skills we have right in front of us that we could use to build a business around.

I worked with Dr. Michelle Flemings, a physician who was responsible for building efficiency into the emergency department (ED) at the hospital where she worked. She managed everything, from monitoring patient turnaround times and huddle meetings with the staff, to making sure departments the ED would interact with like radiology were on the same page with the ED team. She led the team to wait times and turnaround time that other EDs across the country would be envious of.

She developed team-building skills and a wealth of valuable knowledge. The skills she developed were the ones almost every emergency department needs. If she wanted to, could she become a consultant who helped EDs adopt the specific EHR system of her expertise? Absolutely. Alternatively, could she be the consultant who helped EDs become more efficient and consequently more impactful and profitable? Yes.

In Dr. Flemings's case, she had been an ED physician for decades and her goal was to retire from bedside medicine, and she decided to dare her fears and take the leap. She now works with Cerner, a leading EHR company as the lead physician executive and clinical strategist for one of their largest clients.

Finding ways to use your existing skills to change your life is not "pie in the sky" or too good to be true. People like Dr. Flemings prove it most certainly can be done.

These are the kind of things to look for in your own life. Take thirty minutes to do a skills inventory. Look for the skills you picked up before, during, and after your medical training. People are usually shocked by what they discover. Is every skill a pointer to a business you should then go on to start? No. But, it will give you an idea of what options you have available to you.

What do you love and would do for free?

The answer to this can be easy to overlook because you've probably loved it your whole life. To you it feels like common sense; it's simply the air you breathe. But to others it's a valuable skill and something they associate with you.

I realized at some point that this was why I loved EntreMD so much. I've always loved helping people become better versions of themselves. Even when I was a little kid, I would suggest tweaks to people, grown-ups included, on ways they could become better or do something better.

If you get stuck on this one, text a few friends and ask them, "What am I good at? What would you see me doing for free just because I love it so much?" Your friends can help you see obvious things that you don't.

The exercise is very simple but it can be very revealing. You will pick up on trends that you either didn't know about or didn't realize were so obvious to everyone else.

On November 20, 2016, I did this same exercise. I texted five of my friends this question: "What would you say are my unique talents, abilities, or skills?" I was amazed to discover that the answers were very similar.

One friend, Dr. Yaminah Henderson-Fields, listed three things in her response that encapsulated what I was hearing:

1. Being measured in your response to things that others get "worked up" about.

2. Your ability to get others to tap into talents they didn't know they had.

3. Your fidelity to purpose…having a goal, making a plan, and not making excuses.

It shocked me so much that I took a screenshot of it and saved it. (That's how I know the exact date!) It made me pay more attention to these three areas and work hard to develop them further. These are not just "the way I am'." These are gifts I should continue to cultivate so I can serve others to the best of my ability. As I write this, five years after getting that text from my friend, these three things I hope are even more true.

With some reflection, you can find what you love so much you'd do it for free and this could point you to your profitable business idea.

What can you do faster/cheaper/better?

One common block for many doctors in choosing a business idea is the myth that you must have some original idea to succeed in business. These doctors go off in search of a unicorn when there really is no need for it. If you think about it, even if you had an idea as unique as going to space, there are people in the private sector already doing it.

The million-dollar question to ask yourself is can you execute this business idea in a way that is faster or cheaper or better—or maybe all three.

When I launched Ivy League Pediatrics in 2010, there were five other pediatric practices within a ten-minute drive. Why open another practice?

I wanted to do things better. For example, doctor offices are always associated with long wait times. I hated that. I wanted to build a practice where turnaround times were an hour or less, door to door.

I heard many patients complain that they felt like numbers and not people at their doctors' offices. I wanted to build a practice that prioritized warmth and friendliness. I wanted our patients to feel like they were part of a family, the Ivy League Pediatrics family. Did it mean we were not professional? Not at all. Professionalism and warmth can go together.

I also was committed to focus strongly on profitability. Many practices don't, maybe because they think that makes them sound greedy. I see it differently. If a practice goes out of business, everyone loses. Patients lose if they have to be told to find a new doctor. The staff lose their jobs. The community loses out on tax revenue. It's all bad when a practice closes, so I wanted to be focused on profit. Of course patient care comes first but if you want to sustain that, profit can't be far behind.

There's absolutely nothing original about opening a practice. But by doing it faster and better, I was able to be successful.

What makes you sad or mad?

Where there's strong emotion, there's passion. The things that make you sad or mad can be a sure sign of something that can motivate you and fuel a business idea.

For example, I have a student in the EntreMD Business School, Dr. Rebecca Lauderdale, and one of the things that make her both sad and mad is a lack of gender parity for doctors. There are studies that show female physicians making forty to sixty cents on the dollar compared to their male counterparts, performing the exact same things in the exact same specialties. She's building awareness, and consulting with women to show them how to stand up to this unfairness and get what they deserve.

Use these five questions to generate lots of business ideas. Don't worry about having too many. There's no reason to rush the process. You'll be able to pick out the best idea once you have all of them in front of you.

FILTERING YOUR DREAMS THROUGH
THE IDEA MATRIX

As you look at your list of ideas, probably one or two or three will stand out to you. (If it's more than that, work harder to cut it down.)

Now you need to test your top ideas. A business must serve AND earn. Too many people get excited about an idea to serve without putting a lot of thought into how they can earn with it.

Here's a matrix to help you understand the concept:

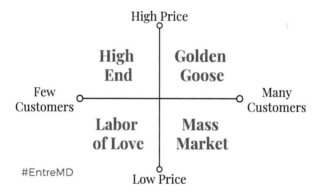

All businesses fall somewhere on this matrix.

The lower right is those businesses that have lots of customers and a low price. Think of Netflix, with plans for around $8 to $10 a month. It's a ridiculously low price, but the company is profitable (to say the least) because they have more than 200 million subscribers. Walmart uses the same model—low prices but a massive customer base. Does this model work? Absolutely. You just need to be clear on the fact that it will require a lot of sales to pull it off.

Above that on the top right is the Golden Goose, where you have both a lot of customers and a high price. iPhones would be a good example of this category. The iPhone 12, for example, sold 100 million units in seven months at $699 per unit. When you do the math, you realize why this category is called the Golden Goose.

Moving to the top left, this is where your high-ticket products and services fall. Think of products like Rolls-Royce or Harley-Davidson or services like a $100,000 coaching or consulting package. With this model you only need a few clients to make significant revenue.

I will stop here to point out something that may not be immediately obvious. You can build a wildly successful business in any of the three quadrants we've looked at so far. Netflix, Apple, and Rolls-Royce are all multiple-billion-dollar companies. Don't let anyone fool you into thinking the only way to do it is high ticket or low ticket. Any of these three will work; you just have to follow the rules.

If you are going to use the low-ticket model, you must be clear that you will have to get a high volume of customers. If you are going to use a high-ticket model, then you must learn to reach a highly qualified audience and offer them a premium product or service. There is no right or wrong. Having said that, don't default to the lower ticket because you're uncomfortable talking about or charging money. Remember, your goal is to become comfortable being uncomfortable.

The only quadrant that must always be avoided is the bottom left. It's not a profitable intersection, and you won't be able to stay in business.

Let's say you have some knowledge of newspaper advertising, and you decide your business will be helping your customers place ads. The problem with this is that the demand for newspaper advertising is now low, and that it's likely to continue trending downward.

So you decided to make your subscription price $49.99 a month. Since that is a low price, you will likely get some takers, but there won't be enough volume (because of the low demand) to keep you in business. This is a classic low demand, low price situation, and exactly what you want to avoid. It's a model that won't become a profitable business.

As you filter your idea through the matrix, try to avoid the tendency to either overestimate or underestimate the amount of people who will want to buy from you.

For example, with EntreMD, it would be easy to take a negative view and say not many doctors want to become entrepreneurs. But then you do the math. There are a million doctors in the US. If only one percent are interested in entrepreneurship, that's still ten thousand doctors. That's plenty to keep me busy.

On the flip side, I could be the wild-eyed dreamer that thinks, wow, there's one million doctors in the US. If I could capture 50 percent of the market, I could make my price ridiculously low and still be amazingly profitable. That's not a realistic assessment, because 50 percent of doctors is a gross overestimation of how many would want to both start their own businesses at this time and work with me.

I have had several clients whose target market is new moms. In 2019, there were 3.75 million births. If 1 percent of new moms would be interested in their product or service, that's still a potential market of 37,500 people to draw from.

I have a client who wants to help women with fibroids.

Small niche, right? Actually, if you pull up the numbers, 80 percent of women say they have fibroids by the time they reach age fifty. Don't make assumptions on the size of your market; do some research.

You might think the biggest problem with doctors and business ideas is talking yourself into a bad idea. That does happen sometimes, but in my experience, the much bigger problem is people talking themselves out of good ideas.

Many struggle to affirm their ideas as valid. All they can see is the caterpillar and envisioning the butterfly is a step too far for them.

This is where I reach back to reading stories of entrepreneurs and also joining a community of entrepreneurs. You realize that every business starts off as a caterpillar, but the stories and community teach you that caterpillars will turn into butterflies.

WHAT DO I DO IF I HAVE TOO MANY IDEAS?

Of course, during your original brainstorming session with the five questions, lots of ideas are a good thing. But if you can't eventually get it down to one great idea, that's a problem.

If you've put your ideas through the matrix and still have more than one idea, I recommend the "magic wand" trick. Imagine holding a magic wand that could automatically make any of these ideas succeed. Which would you choose? That will usually tell you where your heart is and what you'd do for free.

Some people still say, "Can't I just do three ideas?" The answer is no, at least not yet.

Every new business is obscure. You're inside an eggshell, and you have to break out so that people can see you and your business. The only way to do that is to stay hyperfocused on becoming known for one thing.

It's like Beyoncé. She's now known for many businesses—a music streaming service, a film company, clothing line, fragrance line, and other partnerships. She is also a spokesperson for Pepsi and brand ambassador for many brands. But she had to break through in her business and make a name for herself as an artist first.

Concentrate everything on your best business idea first. Eventually you can expand. Choosing to do three businesses at once is like having triplets. All the work involved in the care is tripled. Feed three, change three sets of diapers, put three down for a nap, and on and on. Your businesses will all demand lots of care at the beginning. It won't be an option to say, "I'll give this business one-third of my effort, this business another third, and this business the last third." They all require 100 percent. If you can't make the commitment to perform at 300 percent capacity, I suggest you do them one at a time.

On the opposite end of the spectrum are doctors who tell me they lack ideas. They tried the five questions and didn't get anywhere.

If this is you, remember this. You already own a business; it's called You MD, Inc. You as a physician are a personal brand; you just may not realize it yet. Start building that brand in a way that others can see and then you'll be able to monetize it. I've seen people go on to generate six- and seven-figure revenues on the strength of a personal brand.

What does this look like in practice?

Often there's a topic you're passionate about. Start there. Maybe you're a pediatrician and obesity is your topic. Maybe you're an internal medicine physician who wants to see people fix their lifestyle so they wouldn't have to come see you for chronic disease management. Or possibly you're an OB/GYN and your passion is supporting women in the fourth trimester.

To begin building your personal brand, find ways to speak up and share your knowledge and passion in a way that helps your listeners. You can launch a blog, podcast, or YouTube channel to speak about this consistently. If this sounds too hard, you can start by simply posting about this regularly on social media.

Building a personal brand around your topic can quickly transform into a viable business. The point is don't wait. Right now, you have, or have access to, everything you need to start building. Once you have an audience, you can design products and services to help that audience.

Still stuck? Here's a list of twenty-three business ideas for physicians:

PRIVATE PRACTICE IDEAS

Fee-For-Service

Concierge

Direct Primary Care

Virtual/Telemedicine

Med Spa

PERSONAL BRAND IDEAS

Podcast

Blog

Vlog

Online Courses

MARKETING-BASED IDEAS

Affiliate Marketing

Membership/Subscription

Conference/Retreats

Social Media Influencer

CONSULTING & COACHING IDEAS

Expert Witness

Coaching-Life

Coaching-Career

Coaching-Business

Coaching-Wellness

Medical Expert for TV/Radio

Paid Speaker

CONSUMER PRODUCTS

Skin-Care Line

Apparel

Devices

The main thing is to pick something and get going! It doesn't have to be perfect. Start now. If you get overwhelmed, help is available.

Now that you have an idea, it's time to find out how to connect with the people you can help.

CHAPTER 10

Find Your Message

Everyone is tuned into the same radio station every day, with the call letters WIIFM. Also known as, **What's In It For Me.**

This is how you have to start thinking if you want to be a successful entrepreneur. It doesn't mean you need to start thinking that the whole world is irredeemably selfish or that no one cares about anyone else. That's not true.

But if you want to grab the attention of people, you must work with human nature, not against it. To spark interest and hold it, you must promise there's something in it for us, some reason to care.

I find many new entrepreneurs assume that people will automatically be interested in their message. The cold truth is that nobody's thinking about your message and nobody cares until you give them a reason to. If your goal is to get the opportunity to help people and get rewarded financially for doing it, you need to prove its value in a way they can relate to.

What they do care about is the problem they have, and finding a person who can solve it. If you can discover the problem you solve and articulate it clearly, your success in business becomes inevitable.

Let me make a quick clarification here on terminology. In the world of marketing, the word used for the results you help your customers and clients get is referred to as the "solution." In the world of medicine, we usually talk about patient "outcomes." I have some doctors who, when I say "solution," think of the process used to get to the outcome.

Don't think of the solution as the process; that's not what we want to talk about in our message. We're telling our ideal clients what outcome we are going to get them. In this book, I'm using outcome and solution interchangeably. Please remember that both refer to the person's life after you've solved their problem, not the process you will use to get them there.

THE FOUNDATION OF
YOUR MESSAGE

The foundation of finding your message is actually very simple (which is not the same as saying it's always easy).

You need to clearly define three things:

- Your ideal client.

- The problem they have.

- The outcome you offer.

We're going to dive into the details in a minute but before we do, I'd like to explain why defining these is one of the most important things you can do for your business. When people decide to build a brand around their businesses, they typically start with things like: What's my domain name going to be? What kind of web design do I want? What should my brand colors be?

When it comes to brand building, think of those things as icing on the cake. The actual cake is your message. Your business needs to be known for something. People need to think about your business right away when they have the problem that you solve.

For the message to be obvious to them, it has to be crystal clear to you. Everything in your business should be working together to project what you do and who you do it for. Skipping this step leads to websites that don't grow your business, talks and podcast episodes that don't lead to new customers—the list could go on. Your message is always the starting point of a profitable brand.

Another way to think of this is that you want your business to grow to be a skyscraper, and that requires a deep and wide foundation. And that foundation is always your message. People see all your content, your podcast, your website, and product or services and assume that's your business. They are seeing the part of the skyscraper that is above ground. In truth, it's the focused message that speaks directly to the client's problem and your solution that undergirds the entire building.

Defining Your Ideal Client

Now let's take a closer look at each step in finding your message. First you need to define your ideal client. Some common advice you'll hear on this topic involves creating elaborate avatars with extremely detailed demographic and psychographic information. For most entrepreneurs, this can be very overwhelming and it stops them from going any further.

So my advice is to not get quite that granular, but you still have to be specific. Your ideal client can't be everyone. Defining who you want to talk to is crucial to landing your message. When you talk to everybody, nobody listens.

This lesson came home to me after watching several NBA games. At halftime, the home team often had someone go on the court and chat up the crowd. Pretty much nobody would pay attention. People would munch their popcorn, talk to the person next to them, and pay no attention to what the guy on the court was saying. He was trying to talk to everyone and ended up talking to no one.

Then one halftime, the arena camera focused in on a man about to propose to his girlfriend. You can guess what happened next. The entire arena stopped and listened. He was talking to one person, and suddenly you could hear a pin drop because everyone wanted to listen.

This is why I suggest you think of one person when you create content. Who are you talking to specifically? While I don't think you need detailed demographic information on every aspect of your ideal client to start, you do need to try to think of a specific person, either real or composite, when you communicate with your audience.

What about an ideal client if you're opening a private practice? This will usually be relatively easy to define because you chose an ideal client based on your specialty:

- Women having babies (OB/GYN)

- Parents (Pediatrician)

- People with kidney disease (Nephrologist)

- People with heart disease (Cardiologist)

- Adults with routine or chronic healthcare need (Primary care)

Probably the easiest ideal client to define is when your business is helping people with a problem you yourself overcame. Your ideal client is basically you, but ten years ago (or however long ago it was before you solved your problem).

You know that person's fears. You know their pain, what obstacles will trip them up, what's going to spring up out of nowhere to blindside them. You can talk to them in a way nobody else can because you truly understand what it feels like to be them from the inside.

Your Ideal Client's Problem

Once you have a good definition of your ideal client, you next need to clearly identify the problem they're having. But you must do it in a specific way, and that's from the ideal client's perspective.

Your message needs to resonate with them in a way that makes them instantly say, "Wow, this person understands my problem."

Try this thought experiment. If your ideal client woke up in the middle of the night and started tossing and turning thinking about their problem that you are uniquely able to solve, what are they thinking? Be as specific as possible about the thoughts running through their mind.

This exercise is a great way to avoid being too vague in your messaging. For example, sometimes a student will tell me their message is something like, "I will help you live your best life." People don't wake up in the middle of the night in a sweat thinking, "I'm not living my best life." They think about things like being sick and tired of being in debt, or being alone, or failing as a parent.

It's specific things that keep people up at night, not abstract thoughts. These thoughts are usually articulated by them in simple but powerful ways. Your job is to find those powerful phrases and use them when talking to them.

Let me show you what I mean. For me as a business coach for physicians, my ideal client is me, but a decade ago. When speaking to my ideal client, I could say something like, "I help you learn marketing skills." It's true that you do need marketing skills because that's what can dramatically change the impact your business will have and revenue it will generate.

But I shouldn't lead with that message because that's not how my ideal clients identify their problem. If I'd made the title of this book *How to Market Your Business as a Physician*, would that have been appealing to you? Maybe you would have picked it up but the majority of my audience would not. Why? It doesn't speak to the problem my ideal client is having.

When my ideal clients wake up in the middle of the night in a cold sweat, they are thinking things like:

- I know there's more but I don't know what it is.

- This is not what I imagined my career would look like; where is the freedom?

- I don't have any good business ideas.

- I started a business but I feel like a fraud.
  I have no idea what I'm doing.

- My business isn't making any money.

- I know I need to market but I'm afraid of
  putting myself out there.

- I'm an introvert. I can't network or do talks,
  even though I know it's what I need to do for
  my business to grow.

Now think about how I could flip these problems to podcast episodes. The titles would resonate with my audience because I am speaking their language.

Remember that the whole idea is to find a way to get this down in their words. Think of it like documenting the history of presenting illness (HPI) in a patient's chart. The HPI is supposed to be in the words of your patient, and this is the same idea.

Another way to think of this is that you're joining the conversation your ideal clients are already having in their own heads. It's not about what you want to teach them; it's about what they want to learn. That's the same thing, but the difference in perspective is crucial.

The Outcome You Offer

After defining your ideal client, and getting specific about their problem, it's time to describe your solution in a way your market will understand.

The simplest way to do this is to flip the problem around and promise the opposite.

Here's an example I learned in my pediatric practice. I had many parents tell me, "Dr. Una, I think I'm breaking my child; I really don't know what I'm doing as a parent." Their problem was they had no confidence in their parenting skills. The solution is then obvious: "I'll show you how to parent confidently."

None of this is meant to say that you just say whatever solution they want to hear, whether you can deliver it or not. This all assumes that you can truly help them with their problem. But you must put that solution in words that will resonate with them.

Let's keep going with examples. For weight loss help, it could be as straightforward as, "This program will help you lose weight." Many entrepreneurs have told me they don't say this because that's what everyone says. Well, the reason why everyone says it is because it works!

However, you can dig deeper. The conversation in their heads might be closer to, "Oh my gosh, I can't fit into my skinny jeans anymore. I just let myself go; none of my clothes fit anymore. I can't believe I have to get bigger clothes again."

This means the outcome you offer is: "This program will help you fit into your skinny jeans again." Always think of the problem they are thinking about, and in their own words, and then create the opposite as your solution.

An important part of finding your message is that you always aim to make it as clear as possible. New entrepreneurs often think they need to come up with a clever or cute message. That's not the idea. The goal is for your ideal clients to understand exactly what you're offering. Always choose clear over cute.

When you are clear, your customers don't get confused and then they can say yes to working with you or buying your product. If your message is muddled, they can't get the clarity they need to decide to do business with you.

Let's recall Dr. Yinka from Chapter 9. Her clients repeatedly told her they were concerned with wrinkles and aging skin, but hated the idea of needles and Botox. So her message was the solution to the fears running through their heads. "I help women of color reverse the aging process without pain so they can look a decade younger. If Dr. Yinka tries to generate interest by touting all the technical science behind her line of products, the people who need her services will ignore her, either out of confusion or boredom. Instead, she's successful because she speaks to them from their perspective.

The outcome is always the opposite of the problem, so don't try to reinvent the wheel or get overly creative with some "out of left field" idea. Keep it simple. If the potential client says their problem is, "I can't seem to sleep through the night and I wake up tired," then the solution is the opposite. "Sleep peacefully through the night and wake up refreshed."

PUT ON
YOUR SCIENTIST'S HAT

Once you have a message you think will work, it's time to use that scientific mindset we honed as doctors. Because up till now, your message is like a hypothesis you thought up while sitting in a classroom. Now it's time to head to the lab (the real world) and test your message.

You'll sometimes find your message falls flat. People generally won't tell you that directly. You'll know because you're not getting much response. People ignore it or politely brush it to the side. That's fine. You learned something, and it's time to modify your message.

Other times you'll hit the sweet spot and the response will be enthusiastic. Sometimes during our weekly live sessions in the EntreMD Business School people will type in the chat, "Dr. Una, get out of my head!" That's when I know the message is on target.

Or I'll send out an email and I'll get responses back like, "Oh my goodness, I feel like you wrote this specifically for me. It's exactly what I needed to hear!" This is how dialed in you want to get to your audience's needs.

Learn to listen closely to feedback, because you'll use that skill for as long as you're an entrepreneur. Even after you build an audience and a healthy business income, you'll be listening for messages that hit home and what your audience hungers for. Then you can modify your products and services to solve your ideal clients' problems faster and better. Entrepreneurs listen, and they're always guided by their market.

Please note that I'm not saying to change your business completely with every little bit of feedback you get. A better approach is to stay sensitive to your clients and continually evolve your message to make it better and better.

It helps to be humble on this journey. You'll be deceiving yourself if you think you know your ideal client and their needs deeply enough. Come to the task of discovering who they are with a modest spirit and truly want to get to know them better. Think of yourself as on a quest to discover your ideal clients, because there's always more knowledge and insight available.

This idea of ongoing discovery is also why you should avoid perfectionism in crafting your original message. Create a "good enough" message and get it out there. Test it vigorously, learn, and try again. Rinse and repeat. This is a much more effective method than spending forever trying to come up with a theoretically perfect message.

Of course, this all requires you to encourage your audience to reach out to you in multiple channels. Tell them you want feedback, and then make sure you respond to it.

This lesson was reinforced for me when I launched the EntreMD Business School. The first version of the program was divided into four stages: get clear on your message, amplify your message, define your business model, and define your business systems. I thought that would cover everything my students needed to know.

But then I started seeing comments along the lines of, "I'm not even at stage one yet; I'm still at stage zero because I don't even have a business idea yet!"

This was great feedback. It was my ideal client telling me more about a problem I needed to help them solve. So, we added a stage prior to the other four called stage zero that taught how to find a profitable business idea. Everyone wins when you listen to your audience. They get what they need, and you get happier customers, and more of them.

This formula for finding your message I just outlined works for every kind of business. Coaching, products, mass-market items, service-based, monetizing a personal brand—it doesn't matter what the business is. Because you're always selling a solution.

Why has Geico used the same message for decades? Is there a person left in America who doesn't know that "fifteen minutes could save you 15 percent on car insurance"? I'm sure there must be some, but you get my point. It works because most people's problem with insurance is that it costs too much, but switching companies feels like it will likely be a time-consuming hassle. Geico promises the opposite solution in plain words. This is how business people think because it's been proven to work again and again.

THE MOST COMMON MISTAKE

I want to end this chapter by reemphasizing the priority of finding your message. It must be the first thing after you've found your idea. The most common mistake I see when starting a business is not understanding how fundamental this step is.

- You can build a website, but you must know what message you want on it or it's a waste of time. There is nothing worse than a website that's nothing more than a cute digital business card that does nothing to grow your business.

- You can start a podcast, blog, or YouTube channel but if you haven't defined your main theme (addressing the core problem of your ideal client), the shows will have no focus or the wrong focus. It will end up being an expensive, time-consuming activity with no return on investment.

- Are you buying Facebook ads when you don't know what message you're testing yet? You just wasted a bunch of money. Without a clear message to test, it's like trying to talk to everyone. And remember, when you talk to everyone, no one listens. When you talk to one person, everyone listens.

Understand that this process can be a little messy. Embrace that. Test your message until you get it right, and never be afraid to put something out there and see how your audience reacts.

Your relationship with your ideal clients is analogous to a good marriage. It's sometimes messy, but you lean into that and explore what the other person is like. Do the same for your audience. Make discoveries and be willing to change based on the insights you gather.

Lastly, be strategic in everything you do. How are you weaving your message into all your content? Stay focused. Don't just create content to say, "I created content." You should be testing your message in some form in every piece of content you produce.

Of course, the only way to test your message is to get it out into the world and amplify it. Now, let's look at the final piece of the puzzle.

CHAPTER 11

Amplify Your Message

Y ou know by now that I was lost when it came to marketing when I first opened my pediatric practice in 2010. But I at least knew enough to want to get the name out into the world.

So I reached out to get quotes on television ads. I don't know if you've ever looked into media buys, but the experience was painful for me. First, I'd call up and ask for a quote. Then I'd wait for a few days and finally someone would call me back.

They'd keep me on the phone about an hour explaining a bunch of confusing packages and try to sell me on why they were so great. Then they'd hit me with the prices. I don't remember the exact numbers, but it was way too much for a fledgling practice. Even a small package of measly twenty-second spots was way too much.

So, I thought maybe radio would work. Nope, same experience. I think the cheapest was something like $2,500 for about thirty-five thirty-second spots a month. That's an average of about one spot a day of thirty seconds. I knew I wouldn't get any significant traction from that because the vast majority of the listeners would not be my ideal clients. I would just be wasting money.

I always think about this experience when a coaching client tells me producing consistent content is "too hard."

I tell them, no, it's not. What's too hard is knowing you need to somehow get the word out about your business and feeling like you have no affordable way to do that. I knew I couldn't afford those rates, and there's nothing worse than thinking you have no workable option.

As it turns out, I had more digital marketing options than I knew back then, but that revolution was still in its early stages. There was nowhere near the number of options we have now, and they weren't as easy to navigate as they are now.

Now we live in an age where you can declare that every

Thursday at 1:00 p.m. you're going to do a Facebook Live, call it the Doctor Smith show, and you now have your own TV show with complete control of the content for a grand total of zero dollars. How would you *not* want to take advantage of that opportunity?

That's just scratching the surface. Podcasting is like having your own radio station. The quantity and quality of options available for free or low cost are astounding. Let's be grateful for those resources, and of course, use them!

Just how powerful these tools are came home to me when I started my own Facebook Live show once a week. I called it the Legacy Parent Show and it focused on helping moms and dads learn to parent confidently. People went crazy for it, I got some local celebrity status out of it, and the phone was ringing off the hook at my practice.

The effectiveness of it shocked me. I always ask new families how they found my practice, and I started hearing, "Oh, I watch the Legacy Parent Show so you being our pediatrician was a no-brainer choice."

The results were so overwhelmingly reliable that when I reduced the number of days I saw patients, I also had to stop doing the show because the demand would overwhelm the available appointments.

That's the power of these tools and it's a huge lost opportunity when we don't leverage them. If you take advantage of them, you can establish yourself as a thought leader and expert in your field.

With all these options, if you're hesitating, it likely goes back to the old fear of promoting yourself. You now have the tools to overcome that from previous chapters. Remind yourself that when you don't promote what you do, people who need your solution are stuck with their problem.

You did a lot of work to find your message, now it is time for the next step. Make the decision to amplify your message by putting it on a platform. If nobody hears your message, it's worthless no matter how good it is. You can use these five principles that are easy to follow for amplifying your message.

THE FIVE KEY PRINCIPLES
FOR AMPLIFYING YOUR MESSAGE

Principle 1: Show Up on Your Platform Regularly

Whatever platform channel you choose to use, show up on it frequently, and on a consistent schedule.

When I say platforms, I am referring to YouTube, podcasts, and blogs. I don't include social media because you have a lot less control over who sees your content. (If you're thinking, "Well, I can't do this then because I don't have the time or desire to own a platform," just stay with me. Below I'll tell you how to show up consistently on other platforms without the responsibility of owning one.)

When thinking about a schedule for your platform, I recommend at least weekly. If you're a podcaster, don't do three shows one week, and then go another two weeks without any. Set a time for your episodes to go live each week (or whatever your frequency will be), and then stick to it. Whether it's a YouTube channel or a blog, give your ideal clients fresh content on a regular basis.

Consistency is important for prospective clients to know, like, and trust you. People choose to do business with those they know, like, and trust. When you show up enough times, they'll start to know you. If the content is quality, they'll begin to like you. Then if you prove you can deliver it consistently, and they get results, they'll trust you.

Here's a great example of what I mean. I know a lot of people who are huge consumers of podcasts. If they see a show that sounds interesting to them, the first thing they check is when the last episode was released. If it was a month ago, they're not even going to give that podcast a chance. Why bother if the content is going to be too sporadic? They automatically assume it's not worth subscribing to, and they're probably right.

If you launch a podcast, commit to at least once a week, and then build it into your routine to get it done, no matter what. Make the decision and do it. Please note that having an episode a week doesn't mean you have to record one every week.

One of the secrets that can save a content producer time is batching. For example, I typically record from three to six EntreMD podcasts on my "recording days." That requires one to two hours of my time to do any research and create all the outlines, and then there's the recording time itself.

The beautiful thing about this is that if I record four episodes, that's a month's worth of content. I take multiple four-week breaks from recording episodes of the EntreMD podcast every year but the podcast itself has never been without a new episode every week.

In 2020, I launched my second podcast called Doctors Changing Medicine. I saw that many doctors did not see all the options we have as physicians. Many felt stuck, didn't like their jobs or businesses, but felt their options were limited to a job, a private practice, or being a coach.

I know that the options are endless, so I started this second podcast to solve that problem. My idea for the podcast was to showcase physicians doing things outside the traditional paths.

As much as I loved the idea for a second podcast, I was also worried if it would cause a conflict. The problem for me was that in 2021 I had made it my singular focus to make the EntreMD Business School the number one business school for physicians. I was all in on helping the doctors enrolled get results that far exceeded what they thought was possible for them. I wanted to create a total ecosystem of coaching, accountability, and community.

This new podcast had the potential to take away from that, and I wasn't willing to make that sacrifice.

However, instead of giving up on a second podcast, I decided to take batching to a whole new level. I set apart three days in one month when I would do four to five guest episodes per day. That would give me twelve to fifteen episodes, which was enough content for a quarter.

This is why I don't think you should rule out creating a platform even if you're extremely busy. If you can record in big batches, you can have enough episodes for three months. You could take a whole quarter off as a content creator but still have content going out each week. Batching made it possible for me to launch the Doctors Changing Medicine podcast without sacrificing my commitment to the EntreMD Business School.

Another anxiety I often hear is, "How in the world am I going to keep coming up with ideas for content?" The long answer to that question could fill another book, but I'll give you a short answer that gets to the heart of the matter.

It's impossible to run out of content if you communicate regularly with your ideal clients. They'll ask you questions, and those questions can fuel an endless supply of content. Your content is simply answering those questions.

I use the note-taking app on my phone, and any time I get a question, I answer the person, and then I note the question. When I need to record a podcast episode, I just go to my really long list and choose from there. If you do the same, you'll have a gold mine of content ideas at your fingertips any time.

Beyond questions, you should also pay close attention whenever you and an ideal client are in conversation. They will "off the cuff" share things that you need to pay attention to and can be turned into content:

- **Fears:** What are they and how would you help overcome them?

- **Limiting Beliefs:** What are the most common ones they face that they can't even see?

- **Stories:** Listen for stories of challenges and wins, and then invite them to share them in the form of guest interviews.

When you start looking for it in the right way, you'll quickly see that you can't run out of content.

A bonus tip for this principle: don't just show up on your own platform regularly; show up on the platforms of others as well. This is the best way to put yourself in front of more people who need what you do but have no idea you exist, resulting in a wider audience for you. If someone likes your guest feature, they'll be looking you up for sure. More on this below.

How I put this principle into action: I host two podcasts, releasing three new episodes every week. I also feature on other podcasts at least twice a month.

Principle 2: Include a Call to Action
in Every Piece of Content

I'd say this is the number one mistake of people I see in content creation. There's no call to action to help your audience figure out what to do next.

Your platform is an employee in your business—it's there to work and produce for your business. The platform's job is to spread the word about the pain you fix, and then to help people understand that you're the one with the answer they've been desperately looking for. That's why clear, strong calls to action are an important part of your content.

I have heard people refer to their platforms as passion projects, creative outlets, and labors of love. A blog, YouTube channel, or podcast can be those things. However, if you're an entrepreneur, turning what should be one of the biggest revenue-generating assets in your business into a creative outlet may not be wise.

It's easy for doctors to fall into this trap because we love to teach. (Fun fact: the word doctor comes from the Latin word for teacher.) We do want to primarily teach content in a way to create wins for our audience, but we cannot leave out the call to action.

Leaving out a call to action would be a little like LeBron James dribbling and passing the ball for all four quarters of a game and never taking it to the hoop to score. Dribbling and passing are good and necessary parts of the game, but you have to score if you want to win the game.

Now I want to immediately emphasize there are two primary types of calls to action. The first one is a call to apply what you just taught them. As a new content creator, you may think that people will listen to all the wonderful things you have to teach them, and they will naturally take the next steps to apply what they've learned on their own. The truth is a few will, but most won't unless you tell them what to do. If you give them clear next steps, the chances are much higher that they will take action and create wins for themselves.

The second one is to ask them to work with you. Remember that you serve people at the highest level when they work with you. It is a disservice to not let them know how they can do this.

An example should make this clearer. Let's say I do a podcast and the topic is how and why to launch your own YouTube channel. My call to action will be to tell the members of my audience to set a date to launch their own YouTube channel. I spent the show telling them the why and the how of it, and now I give them a concrete action to execute.

Here's another example. If I do a show with advice on launching their own podcast, my call to action could be for them to reach out to three potential guests that week. Give your audience these kinds of actions each week and it will change their lives in ways both big and small.

You might be surprised by the impact a regular call to action makes. Many people will listen to a show and love it, but if you don't give them an action, they often do nothing. But if you specify what they should do, a lot of people will do it.

Your audience will appreciate it. A doctor left me a review and said that her private practice survived the pandemic because of my podcast. What if I hadn't given her calls to action? If you want to make a difference with people, you've got to teach them, but also tell them what to do next.

What about a call to action to do business with you—should you do that? Yes. I recommend that when you deliver an amazing piece of content, say something along these lines:

> Thank you for listening to this episode. I know you found it to be very helpful. If you're tired of [insert pain points] and you're ready for [insert outcome], come work with me. Go to www.yourprogram.com to sign up. I'm looking forward to it!

Your call to action should be strong, never wimpy. The example above is a strong call to action. I have heard many weak ones at the end of a YouTube video or podcast episode. "If you want more information about what I do, you can check it out on my website."

No one wants more information. They have a pain, they want it gone, and they want to know if you're the person for the job. So you tell them they have a pain, you tell them you can solve it, and you tell them how they can sign up. Do you see the difference?

Don't feel sleazy; don't feel weird. I hope by this point in the book you've accepted your value and realize that your clients get the highest level of service when they work directly with you.

Bonus tip: you can do a combination call to action that includes one task for your audience, and one call to sign up to work with you. Here's what that would look like.

Let's say you create a video on the seven types of social media posts. The double call to action would sound something like this:

Now I want you to decide how many days a week you're going to post on social media and which types of posts you'll use. That's your action for this week. And if you want to become great at promoting your business so it creates financial freedom for you, come join us in the EntreMD Business School. It is the only school of its kind exclusively for physicians who want to thrive as entrepreneurs. Go to www.entremd.com/business to save your spot.

Do you see how neatly that fits together? There's no pressure or sleazy tactics. It just gives your audience options.

Content creation takes a ton of time. If you're not doing it intentionally and strategically, it's a lot of time spent on something that does not move the needle in your business. Doing it this way ensures that every piece of content works hard to generate more patients and/or clients for you.

How I put this principle into action: I have a rule to never publish content without a call to action.

Principle 3: Cast a Wide Net

Creating lots of great content is step one. But you must spread the word, too, or it won't get near the audience it should. Don't just create a new YouTube video and leave it at that;

tease it and post links to it from your social media accounts. Tell your mailing list you created a new video and link to it. Remind people who see the video to subscribe to your YouTube channel.

When you speak at events, tell them about your platform. When you talk to people one-on-one, tell them too. Describe a little about what you do on your platforms and how often you release content. Let them know the problem your platform solves and the outcomes it creates, and they won't be able to resist looking it up.

Here's what that would look like. When chatting with an ideal client one-on-one, answer any specific question they have, and then direct them to a piece of content for more. "That's the short answer. If you want to go deeper, you should really listen to the podcast episode I did on this same topic. You can find it…"

Also, don't just cast a wide net. Keep throwing the net out there repeatedly. When you promote each piece of content, you're also promoting your business. How? Remember the call to action. Every piece of content creates wins for your ideal clients and gives them reasons why they need to work with you. All that effort will add up and work like compound interest. It can be astonishing to watch your business grow exponentially as these efforts begin snowballing.

The widest possible net—the granddaddy of promoting your content, if you will—is to be a guest on other people's platforms. You're accessing their entire audience, and on top of that the host is lending you his or her credibility. That's a huge advantage and can expose you to larger numbers of other people. Be sure to actively seek guest spots.

Lastly, casting a wide net only works when you consistently produce good content. Good means it is true to your message and it solves problems. Set a schedule for these and take all the "only if I feel like it" out of the equation.

How I put this principle into action: This is how I distribute every single podcast episode, every single week.

- Two emails every week to announce the episodes

- Two dedicated social media posts to announce the episodes

- Speak at events quarterly

- Guest on two podcasts a month (I'll call myself out real quick because this should be four!)

- Share the podcast episodes in the EntreMD Business School

- Share specific episodes when people ask me questions 1:1

Principle 4: Be Disciplined in Your Messaging

This is about staying true to your ideal clients. If you really want to help them, you need to keep your content squarely focused on addressing their pain and giving them a solution. On the EntreMD Podcast, for instance, my job is to keep helping my listeners create wins as entrepreneurs. I focus on answering their questions, discerning fear and limiting beliefs, and helping them overcome those. I look for ways to help them elevate their belief in themselves.

I see too many entrepreneurs get a bad case of "squirrelitis," as I like to call it. They're darting off everywhere. "I can teach them how to start a business. I could show them how to invest in real estate too. I just celebrated my twenty-fifth wedding anniversary, so I have a lot to teach them on marriage too. When I think of it, I have too much to offer. I don't want to help one kind of client. I actually have four ideal clients."

When you jump all over the place, people won't know why they're coming to your platform. It erodes your authority. They start wondering, "What is this person actually an expert on?" Your audience needs to know why they're coming to you, and that they can trust you'll deliver it consistently.

It's fine to love a lot of things, but if you want to have a big impact, focus on one thing and stay on message. Does this mean you can never talk about anything else? No, it doesn't.

For instance, episode #143 of the EntreMD podcast is titled, "Entrepreneurship for Parents of Young Kids." This is a little off my main focus, because it's not directly about how-to's in business. However, it does address a pain point for many of my ideal clients.

The question had come up many times in the EntreMD private Facebook group and it was creating hiccups for some of my students' businesses. So I address it in one podcast episode, but I would not create a course on it or a signature talk about it. The topic is relevant, but not central to my audience's problem.

The best way to think about staying disciplined is to remind yourself that your platform is not for you. It's to serve your ideal client. If you remember that, it will keep you disciplined and on message. Staying focused can be the difference between a meandering business that never makes any real impact or money and a seven-figure powerhouse.

How I put this principle into action: On my EntreMD podcast, I only speak to physician entrepreneurs and I only deliver content that will help them thrive as entrepreneurs.

Principle 5: Everything Needs to Be a Win–Win

This last principle is like a summary of all the previous principles. The goal of every piece of content should be a win for the people who consume it, and a win for you.

Think back to biology class and the lessons on parasitic relationships, where one organism gets its nutrients at the expense of another organism. You never want to be that organism in the business world, whether it's as the host or the parasite. You want to create symbiotic relationships that are mutually beneficial.

All your content should have value for your ideal client. That's their win. If it doesn't have value to them and they don't get regular wins from it, they'll forget about you.

But you also need to think about how a piece of content will advance your business. How will it get clients for you? Is every piece of content centered around the problem–solution message at the heart of your business? Everything you do needs to advance the ball in the direction of engaging with ideal clients and getting them to know, like, and trust you. When you do that, it will be easy for them to say yes to your products and services.

How I put this principle into action: Before producing a piece of content, I define what I want my listeners to get out of it and what I want to get out of it. This way, my content is intentionally curated to create the desired outcome.

IF YOU DON'T WANT TO LAUNCH A PLATFORM YET

Maybe you don't want to take on the task of starting a blog, podcast, or YouTube channel.

Don't let that stop you from amplifying your voice. You could choose to be a guest on someone else's platform four times a month for instance. That would add up to putting yourself out there an average of once a week. You'll be publishing as frequently as any consistent content creator out there.

You might think you will be bothering people. Remember that if there is anything an interview show needs, it's guests. You'll be helping, not bothering them.

IT'S TIME TO TAKE YOUR OWN JOURNEY WITH THE ENTREMD METHOD

All of these steps might feel a little overwhelming as you think about implementing the EntreMD Method. It's actually easier than you think to take control and gain your freedom. The key is to remember the fundamentals:

- Overcome the mindset myths

- Change your habits

- Discover and own your business idea

- Tell as many people as possible what you do

- Invite them directly to work with you

You will be well on your way to creating a successful business.

This formula has been used by over a hundred doctors over the last three years and many have gone on to create six-, multiple-six-, and seven-figure businesses. You now have your proven roadmap that will ultimately lead to financial freedom and the ability to live life and practice medicine on your terms. Now let's wrap it up and remind you of what you need to do next.

Conclusion

I wanted to tell you a small but important story to conclude the journey of this book. You might recall the story of my first live event for EntreMD in 2019. The hotel I originally wanted was too expensive, I was worried I wasn't ready, and I didn't know if anybody would come. But I decided to do it anyway.

Dr. Chiagozie Fawole, Founder of SavvyDocs in Real Estate, attended that first ever event. Two years later, she sent out an email encouraging her audience to attend the next live event. Her subject line was: "One event that changed everything" and this is in part what she said:

"In June 2019, I took a flight down to Atlanta to attend the first EntreMD Live. I had spoken with Dr. Una on the phone about how medicine was changing, and just KNEW I had to connect with her in person. Turns out, that event would ignite something much bigger in me, and now, two years later, this introverted introvert has come out of her shell."

Dr. Fawole went on to list a bunch of accomplishments, including cutting back on her time at work and launching a business to help physicians invest in real estate.

At the time of this writing, she has cut back her hours at work by half (0.5 FTE), and crossed the six-figure-a-year milestone in her business.

My favorite thing about this email is thinking about what would've happened if I'd given into my fears. The change for Dr. Fawole might never have happened. There are many other success stories from my work, some smaller, some bigger. But sometimes I like to reflect on the sum total of impacts we can make in the world when we have the courage to move forward with our dreams. Every story counts.

It's genuinely a privilege to impact lives in ways that change them permanently. It's ultimately why I do what I do, and why I always say I've never had to work a day in EntreMD. It's just way too much fun to call work.

You can be in the business of changing lives, too, in ways both big and small. That's really what's at stake here, and what keeps us motivated.

Take a moment to think of what will be possible in the lives of others if you say yes to your dreams and start this journey. It could be an extra day off each week to spend with the kids. Or it could be being able to hire a scribe to take your notes so you always get home on time to be present to your spouse. It might even lead to a seven-figure business that allows you to give a $100,000 donation to your favorite charity. Think of all the possibilities.

Of course, the greatest reward for going on this journey is not what you create, impressive as that will be. It is who you become in the process.

WHAT TO DO NEXT

Start Taking Action Today

This is one of the superpowers of the ultrasuccessful. Don't wait. Tomorrow is not a better day than today. Your action could be as "little" as adopting the five daily habits introduced in Chapter 6 or as "big" as putting in an offer for an office building. Take your next step and commit to doing that over and over and over again. You have what you need to take back control of your career and life right here in this book.

Continue Your Business Education

The EntreMD Podcast is the place where I show up weekly to inspire you and give you actionable steps on your journey. Think of it as continuing business education (CBE), not unlike our continuing medical education (CME). I release two episodes every single week. The conversation doesn't need to end here.

Take the Leap

If the EntreMD method resonates with you but you know you would thrive if you were doing this in a community of physician entrepreneurs who are committed to the method, come join us in the EntreMD Business School.

AND MOST OF ALL...

Don't wait for perfection. Aim for excellence and then take action. Don't be afraid to act or ask for help on your journey.

I'm rooting for you, always!

Acknowledgments

I want to thank the following special people:

My husband, Steve: for being my mentor, greatest cheerleader, and fan. You taught me to dream big, take bold steps, and never take no for an answer. I couldn't have done this without you.

My four kids, Cheta, Chidi, Chichi, and Esther: for inspiring me every day to be the best version of myself.

My executive assistant, Makeda: for taking a lot off my plate so I have the freedom to live nine lives at once.

The EntreMD community, and especially the doctors in the EntreMD Business School: for the honor and privilege of serving you and helping you create careers, businesses, and lives that are nothing short of magical.

About the Author

DR. NNEKA UNACHUKWU is a board-certified pediatrician and the Founder and CEO of Ivy League Pediatrics outside of Atlanta, Georgia. She graduated from the University of Nigeria College of Medicine and completed her residency in New Jersey before opening her own practice.

Fondly known as **DR. UNA**, she founded EntreMD in response to drastic shifts for doctors in the healthcare field, including loss of autonomy, job insecurity, and unparalleled dissatisfaction. The mission of EntreMD is to help doctors build profitable businesses so they can live life and practice medicine on their own terms. Her popular offerings include the EntreMD Business School, live events, and the EntreMD Podcast. The podcast is listened to in over one hundred countries and has exceeded 150,000 downloads in less than two years. She is a highly sought-after speaker, a regular contributor to *Forbes*, and a member of the Forbes Business Council.